Physical Fitness: The Water Aerobics Way

Terry-Ann Spitzer
Werner W.K. Hoeger
Boise State University

Morton Publishing Company
925 W. Kenyon Ave., Unit 12
Englewood, Colorado 80110

This book is dedicated to my mom and in memory of my dad.

— Terry-Ann Spitzer

The authors wish to thank all of those who so graciously donated their time and efforts to make this work possible. Sharon A. Hoeger for her valuable input and suggestions in he preparation of the final manuscript; Charles B. Scheer for the cover photographs; Dr. Glenn Potter for his support and encouragement; and Rachel Banashek, Cherianne Calkins, Chrissy Koennecker, Anne Staker, and Eric LaMott for their help with the photography in this book.

Printed in the United States of America

10 9 8 7 6 5 4 3 2

ISBN: 0-89582-206-7

Preface

More than ever before Americans realize that good health is largely self-controlled and that premature illness and mortality can be prevented through adequate fitness and positive lifestyle habits. Recent scientific research indicates that active people live longer and enjoy a better quality of life. As a result, the importance of sound physical fitness programs has taken an entire new dimension. From an initial fitness fad in the early 1970s, fitness programs have become a trend that is now very much a part of the American way of life.

Unfortunately many popular "land-based" fitness activities, such as jogging and aerobic dance, are contraindicated for people with selected muscular-skeletal problems. Most land-based activities place a tremendous amount of stress on joints, ligaments, bones, tendons, and muscles, and over half of all new participants drop out within the first six weeks due to injuries.

In the quest for the "ideal" fitness activity, an ever increasing number of fitness participants are discovering water aerobics as the perfect alternative to traditional land-based programs. Water aerobics provides fitness, fun, and safety for people of all ages, with virtually no impact (no risk of injury) to the muscular or skeletal systems. Aquatic exercise has become one of the fastest growing fitness activities in the United States. From an initial 200,000 participants in 1983, approximately 2.5 million people were participating in 1989. Most experts anticipate that this trend will continue to increase by leaps and bounds over the next decade.

This book, *Physical Fitness: The Water Aerobics Way*, has been written as a text for water aerobic fitness classes or programs at colleges and universities, health/fitness clubs, and health promotion programs in general. Since most theoretical information is often overlooked, the use of this book will provide an excellent resource guide to all participants.

As the title indicates, *Physical Fitness: The Water Aerobics Way*, discusses how fitness can be achieved safely and effectively through a water aerobics program. The text also addresses a healthy lifestyle program that if implemented, will help the participant enjoy a healthier, happier, and more productive life.

Table of Contents

1 • Why Fitness: The Water Aerobics Way? 1

2 • Physical Fitness: Components and Assessment 9

3 • Water Aerobics Fitness Program 33

Exercise Tips 60

Exercises 1–88 61

4 • Nutrition and Weight Control 111

5 • A Healthy Lifestyle Approach 131

APPENDIX A • Health History Questionnaire 145

APPENDIX B • Personal Fitness Profile: Pre-Test 147

Personal Fitness Profile: Post Test 148

References 149

Index 151

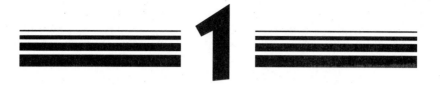

Why Fitness: The Water Aerobics Way?

Most people in the United States would like to enjoy physical fitness and total well-being. As a result, from an initial fitness fad in the early 1970s, fitness programs have become a trend that is now very much a part of the American way of life. The increase in the number of fitness participants is attributed primarily to scientific evidence linking vigorous exercise and positive lifestyle habits to better health and improved quality of life.

Many research findings have shown that physical inactivity and negative lifestyle habits are a serious threat to an individual's health. Movement and activity are basic functions needed by the human organism to grow, develop, and maintain health. However, the automated society in which we live no longer provides the body with sufficient activity to insure good health, but rather increases the deterioration rate of the human body. While medical advances have virtually eliminated infectious diseases, the so-called "good life" (sedentary living, alcohol, fatty foods, excessive sweets, tobacco, drugs, etc.) has brought about increases in the incidence of chronic diseases such as hypertension, coronary heart disease, and strokes.

As chronic diseases increased, it became clear that prevention was the best medicine. People began to realize that good health is largely self-controlled and that premature deaths and illnesses could be prevented through adherence to fitness programs and positive lifestyle habits.

PHYSICAL FITNESS

The American Medical Association defines fitness as the general capacity to adapt and respond favorably to physical effort. This implies that individuals are physically fit when they can meet ordinary as well as the unusual demands of daily life, safely and effectively without being over fatigued and still have energy left for leisure and recreational activities. From a health standpoint, physical fitness has four major components:

1. Cardiovascular endurance — defined as the ability of the heart, lungs, and blood vessels to supply oxygen and nutrients to the muscles for sustained exercise.
2. Muscular strength and endurance — which refers to the ability of the muscles to generate force.
3. Flexibility — defined as the capacity of a joint to move freely through a full range of motion.

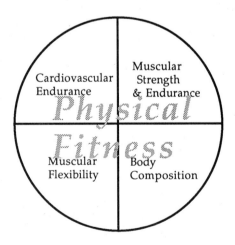

FIGURE 1.1. Health-Related components of physical fitness.

4. Body composition — used in reference to the amount of lean body mass and adipose tissue (fat mass) found in the human body.

A well designed fitness program will not only contribute to the development of these four fitness components, but will also provide many other health benefits. Additional benefits will be discussed throughout the book. Without question, however, an improvement in the quality of life is the greatest benefit that any fitness program will provide to the habitual participant.

WATER AEROBICS

Water aerobics is one of the most invigorating fitness activities presently available. Some very simple words best describe this new form of exercise: fitness, fun, and safety for all people of all ages. A well-designed water aerobics program: (a) helps develop the various components of fitness, (b) provides an opportunity for socialization and fun in a very comfortable and refreshing setting, and (c) provides a relatively safe environment for injury-free exercise participation.

The aquatic exercises used during water aerobics are designed to elevate the heart rate, which contributes to cardiovascular development; provide increased resistance for strength improvement with virtually no impact; help the joints move through their range of motion, thereby promoting flexibility; and facilitate weight reduction without the "pain" and fear of injuries experienced by many individuals who initiate exercise programs. Additionally, water aerobics is an activity available to swimmers and non-swimmers alike because most exercises are conducted while standing in armpit deep water or while holding on to some other form of support.

The nationwide popularity of aquatic exercise has increased from about 200,000 participants in 1983 to approximately 2.5 million in 1990. Water aerobics has certainly become a popular alternative to traditional forms of fitness programs and has gained recognition and respect from all segments of the fitness and wellness movement across America.

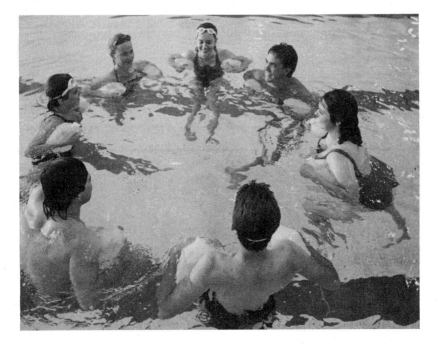

FIGURE 1.2. Water Aerobics: One of the fastest growing fitness activities in America.

Swimmers have known for decades about the benefits of exercise in an aquatic environment. Water aerobics, however, has only been promoted as a fitness activity in the past few years. While swimming for cardiovascular development is limited to highly skilled individuals, water aerobics opens up aquatic exercise to all ability levels. Track coaches and physical therapists were among the first to recognize the potential of aquatic exercises in a vertical position. Injured athletes and other patients were often sent to a pool for rehabilitation. In this type of environment, they could still exercise to maintain cardiovascular endurance and yet limit the potential for further injury.

Advantages of Water Aerobics

Because of the aquatic environment, water aerobics provides tremendous advantages over traditional forms of fitness activities.

The exercise program can be individualized and adapted to fit all kinds of needs and abilities. The resistance of the water will challenge beginners as well as highly-conditioned athletes. Furthermore, the water provides a cushioned environment to help decrease the risk of injuries and at the same time it is an excellent exercise alternative for people with a wide range of joint problems. These characteristics make water aerobics a unique fitness activity suitable for a greater percentage of the population.

For many fitness participants, finding the ideal activity to develop the various components of fitness, without causing injury, has been difficult. According to some reports, approximately 60 percent of the people who begin an exercise program will drop out in the initial six weeks due to injuries. Because we live in a world of gravity, striking activities such as jogging and aerobic dance can place tremendous stress on joints, bones, tendons, and ligaments. Overuse injuries are especially common among beginners who choose such types of exercise. Activities that involve excessive pounding or jarring have to be reduced for individuals with joint problems or arthritis, the elderly, or those who are obese. This in turn limits the kinds of fitness activities available to them.

Water, however, provides a media where jarring can be limited. Water is 1,000 times more dense than air, and therefore it provides buoyancy to most objects immersed therein. Because of this buoyancy, the human body weighs much less in water, creating a cushioning effect that places much less stress on the body.

The enhancement of muscular endurance in water aerobics is superior to most land-based fitness activities. The increased density of water creates a greater resistance, which in turn provides a heavier workload for the active muscle groups. This increased workload better stimulates muscular development and enhances toning.

Another advantage of water aerobics is that it requires upper and lower extremity work, thereby making it a total body workout. Activities such as jogging and walking do little to improve the condition of the upper body. Water aerobics, on the other hand, combines locomotor and jumping exercises to develop the lower extremities with resistance exercises for the upper extremities.

Water aerobics also provides a cooler and more comfortable climate in which to exercise. Exercising muscles produce heat as a by-product of energy metabolism which in turn increases body temperature. Many individuals, especially those who are obese, are not heat tolerant and therefore are unable to exercise in warm temperatures. Heat can be dissipated much more efficiently in water than on land. Consequently, aquatic exercise significantly reduces heat stress and makes exercise more comfortable and invigorating. Heat stroke and heat exhaustion illness are virtually eliminated in water aerobics (except when water temperatures are kept abnormally high).

A distinctive advantage of water aerobic exercises is that they do not require large areas of space. If you can stand in water up to your chest (armpit level), have a smooth and uniform bottom surface, and three to four feet of free space around you, the exercises can be easily performed.

Water also provides an anonymous environment in which to exercise. It is difficult to see details in water. Many individuals are uncomfortable with exercising in public and for them water aerobics is the answer.

With water aerobics you do not have to be highly skilled to gain fitness benefits. Since most exercises are done while standing in armpit water level, even non-swimmers, with lifeguard supervision, can participate.

Benefits of a Water Aerobics Fitness Program

While it is difficult to compile an all-inclusive list of the benefits that you can expect from regular participation in a water aerobics fitness program, the following list will provide a summary of some of the benefits.

1. Improves and strengthens the cardiovascular system (improves oxygen supply to all parts of the body, including the heart, muscles, and the brain).
2. Improves muscular tone, muscular strength, and muscular endurance.
3. Improves muscular flexibility.
4. Helps maintain ideal body weight.
5. Improves posture and physical appearance.

6. Decreases the risk for chronic diseases and illnesses (heart disease, stroke, high blood pressure, pulmonary disease, arthritis, etc.).
7. Relieves tension and helps in coping with stresses of life.
8. Increases levels of energy and job productivity.
9. Slows down the aging process.
10. Improves self-image and morale and aids in fighting depression.
11. Motivates toward positive lifestyle changes (better nutrition, smoking cessation, alcohol and drug abuse control).
12. Decreases recovery time following physical exertion.
13. Speeds up recovery following injury and/or disease.
14. Regulates and improves overall body functions.
15. Eases the process of childbearing and childbirth.
16. Improves the quality of life.

While there are many advantages and benefits to be derived through regular participation in a well-designed water aerobics exercise program, little literature is currently available on this relatively new fitness activity. In this regard, the information presented in the next four chapters has been written not only to provide the reader with all of the necessary guidelines to develop a sound water aerobics exercise program, but also to implement a lifetime program to improve physical fitness and promote personal wellness. Keep in mind that good fitness and positive lifestyle practices will greatly contribute toward the enhancement and maintenance of good health. You are encouraged to be persistent and committed because only you can take control of your lifestyle and thereby reap the benefits of wellness.

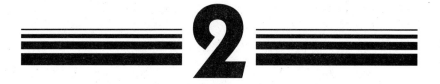

Physical Fitness: Components And Assessment

In this chapter the four health-related components of physical fitness will be discussed and techniques used in their assessment will be described. You can use these tests regularly to assess improvements in fitness as you engage in your exercise program. You are encouraged to take these tests at least once as you begin your exercise program and later repeat the assessments after eight to twelve weeks of exercise participation. You may record the results of your fitness assessments on the forms provided in Appendix B.

   Exercise testing and/or exercise participation is contraindicated for individuals with certain medical or physical conditions. Therefore, before you start a water exercise program or participate in any exercise testing, fill out the health history questionnaire given in Appendix A. If your answer to any of the questions is positive, consult your doctor before initiating, continuing, or increasing your level of physical activity.

CARDIOVASCULAR ENDURANCE ASSESSMENT

Cardiovascular endurance, cardiovascular fitness, or aerobic capacity has been defined as the ability of the lungs, heart, and blood vessels to deliver adequate amounts of oxygen and nutrients to the cells to meet the demands of prolonged physical activity. As a person breathes, part of the oxygen contained in ambient air is taken up in the lungs and transported in the blood to the heart. The heart is then responsible for pumping the oxygenated blood through the circulatory system to all organs and tissues of the body. At the cellular level, oxygen is used to convert food substrates, primarily carbohydrates and fats, into energy necessary to conduct body functions and maintain a constant internal equilibrium.

A sound cardiovascular endurance program greatly contributes toward the enhancement and maintenance of good health. The "typical" American is not exactly a good role model when it comes to physical fitness. A poorly conditioned heart which has to pump more often just to keep a person alive is subject to more wear-and-tear than a well-conditioned heart. In situations where strenuous demands are placed on the heart, such as doing yard work, lifting heavy objects or weights, or running to catch a train, the unconditioned heart may not be able to sustain the strain.

Every individual who initiates a cardiovascular exercise program can expect a number of benefits that result from training. Among these benefits are a decrease in resting heart rate, blood pressure, blood lipids (cholesterol and triglycerides), recovery time following exercise, and risk for hypokinetic diseases (those associated with physical inactivity and sedentary living). There is also an increase in cardiac muscle strength and oxygen carrying capacity in the body.

Cardiovascular endurance is determined by the maximal amount of oxygen that the human body is able to utilize per minute of physical activity. This value is commonly expressed in milliliters of oxygen per kilogram of body weight per minute of physical activity (ml/kg/min). Since all tissues and organs of the body utilize oxygen to function, a higher amount of oxygen consumption indicates a more efficient cardiovascular system.

During physical exertion, a greater amount of energy is needed to carry out the work. As a result, the heart, lungs, and blood vessels have to deliver more oxygen to the cells to supply the required energy to accomplish the task. During prolonged physical activity, an individual with a high level of cardiovascular endurance is able to deliver the required amount of oxygen to the tissues with relative ease. The cardiovascular system of a person with a low level of endurance would have to work much harder, since the heart would have to pump more often to supply the same amount of oxygen to the tissues, and consequently would fatigue faster. Hence, a higher capacity to deliver and utilize oxygen (oxygen uptake) indicates a more efficient cardiovascular system.

The most frequently used test to determine cardiovascular fitness is the 1.5-mile run/walk test. Your fitness category is determined according to the time it takes to run/walk a 1.5-mile course. The only equipment necessary to conduct this test is a stopwatch and a track or premeasured 1.5-mile course.

It is a very simple test to administer, but caution should be taken when conducting the test. Since the objective of the test is to cover the distance in the shortest period of time, the use of this test should be limited to conditioned individuals who have been cleared for exercise. It is contraindicated for unconditioned beginners (you should have at least six weeks of aerobic training), symptomatic individuals, and those with known cardiovascular disease and/or heart disease risk factors. If medical clearance is necessary (see Appendix A) or you have any questions regarding your ability to safely participate in an exercise program, you should check with a physician before you take the test.

Prior to taking the 1.5-mile run/walk test you should conduct a few warm-up exercises. Do some stretching exercises, some walking, and slow jogging. Next, time yourself during the run/walk to see how fast you cover the distance. If any unusual symptoms arise during the test, do not continue. Stop immediately, see your physician and/or retake the test after another six weeks of aerobic training. At the end of the test, cool down by walking or jogging slowly for another three to five minutes. According to your performance time, look up your estimated maximal oxygen uptake in Table 2.1 and your corresponding fitness category in Table 2.2.

For example, a 20-year-old female runs the 1.5-mile course in 12 minutes and 40 seconds. Table 2.1 shows a maximal oxygen uptake of 39.8 ml/kg/min for a time of 12:40. According to Table

TABLE 2.1.

Estimated Maximal Oxygen Uptake in ml/kg/min for the 1.5-Mile Run Test

Time	Max VO₂	Time	Max VO₂	Time	Max VO₂	Time	Max VO₂	Time	Max VO₂
6:10	80.0	8:50	59.1	11:30	44.4	14:10	35.5	16:50	29.1
6:20	79.0	9:00	58.1	11:40	43.7	14:20	35.1	17:00	28.9
6:30	77.9	9:10	56.9	11:50	43.2	14:30	34.7	17:10	28.5
6:40	76.7	9:20	55.9	12:00	42.3	14:40	34.3	17:20	28.3
6:50	75.5	9:30	54.7	12:10	41.7	14:50	34.0	17:30	28.0
7:00	74.0	9:40	53.5	12:20	41.0	15:00	33.6	17:40	27.7
7:10	72.6	9:50	52.3	12:30	40.4	15:10	33.1	17:50	27.4
7:20	71.3	10:00	51.1	12:40	39.8	15:20	32.7	18:00	27.1
7:30	69.9	10:10	50.4	12:50	39.2	15:30	32.2	18:10	26.8
7:40	68.3	10:20	49.5	13:00	38.6	15:40	31.8	18:20	26.6
7:50	66.8	10:30	48.6	13:10	38.1	15:50	31.4	18:30	26.3
8:00	65.2	10:40	48.0	13:20	37.8	16:00	30.9	18:40	26.0
8:10	63.9	10:50	47.4	13:30	37.2	16:10	30.5	18:50	25.7
8:20	62.5	11:00	46.6	13:40	36.8	16:20	30.2	19:00	25.4
8:30	61.2	11:10	45.8	13:50	36.3	16:30	29.8		
8:40	60.2	11:20	45.1	14:00	35.9	16:40	29.5		

Adapted from Cooper, K. H. "A Means of Assessing Maximal Oxygen Intake." *JAMA* 203:201–204, 1968; Pollock, M. L. et al. *Health and Fitness Through Physical Activity*. New York: John Wiley and Sons, 1978; Wilmore, H. J. *Training for Sport and Activity*. Boston: Allyn and Bacon, 1982.

TABLE 2.2.

Cardiovascular Fitness Classification According to
Maximal Oxygen Uptake in ml/kg/min

Sex	Age	Fitness Classification				
		Poor	Fair	Average	Good*	Excellent
Men	<29	<25	25-33	34-42	43-52	53+
	30-39	<23	23-30	31-38	39-48	49+
	40-49	<20	20-26	27-35	36-44	45+
	50-59	<18	18-24	25-33	34-42	43+
	60-69	<16	16-22	23-30	31-40	41+
Women	<29	<24	24-30	31-37	38-48	49+
	30-39	<20	20-27	28-33	34-44	45+
	40-49	<17	17-23	24-30	31-41	42+
	50-59	<15	15-20	21-27	28-37	38+
	60-69	<13	13-17	18-23	24-34	35+

*Recommended health-fitness standard

2.2, this maximal oxygen uptake would place her in the good cardiovascular fitness category.

MUSCULAR STRENGTH/ENDURANCE ASSESSMENT

Many people are under the impression that muscular strength and endurance are only necessary for athletes and other individuals who hold jobs that require heavy muscular work. However, strength and endurance are important components of total physical fitness and have become an integral part of everyone's life.

Adequate levels of strength significantly enhance a person's health and well-being throughout life. Strength is crucial for optimal performance in daily activities such as sitting, walking, running, lifting and carrying objects, doing housework, or even for the enjoyment of recreational activities. Strength is also of great value in improving personal appearance and self-image, in developing sports skills, and in meeting certain emergencies in life where strength is necessary to cope effectively.

Perhaps one of the most significant benefits of maintaining a good strength level is its relationship to human metabolism. Metabolism is defined as all energy and material transformations that occur within living cells. Several studies have shown that there is a relationship between oxygen consumption as a result of metabolic activity and amount of lean body mass.

Muscle tissue uses energy even at rest, while fatty tissue uses very little energy and may be considered metabolically inert from the point of view of caloric use. As muscle size increases, so does the resting metabolism or the amount of energy (expressed in calories) required by an individual during resting conditions to sustain proper cell function. Even small increases in muscle mass increase resting metabolism.

Estimates indicate that each additional pound of muscle tissue increases resting metabolism by 50 to 100 calories per day. All other factors being equal, if one takes two individuals at 150 pounds with different amounts of muscle mass, let's say five pounds, the one with the greater muscle mass will have a higher resting metabolic rate, allowing this person to eat more calories to maintain the muscle tissue.

Although muscular strength and endurance are interrelated, a basic difference exists between the two. Strength is defined as the ability to exert maximum force against resistance. Endurance is the ability of a muscle to exert submaximal force repeatedly over a period of time. Muscular endurance depends to a large extent on muscular strength and to a lesser extent on cardiovascular endurance. Weak muscles cannot repeat an action several times, nor sustain it for a prolonged period of time.

Muscular strength is usually determined by the maximal amount of resistance (one repetition maximum or 1 RM) that an individual is able to lift in a single effort. This assessment gives a good measure of absolute strength, but it does require a considerable amount of time to administer. Muscular endurance is commonly established by the number of repetitions that an individual can perform against a submaximal resistance or by the length of time that a given contraction can be sustained.

Because water aerobics contributes primarily to the development of muscular endurance, a muscular endurance test has been selected to determine your strength level. Three exercises have been selected for your muscular endurance test. These exercises will help assess the endurance of the upper body, lower body, and abdominal muscle groups. You will only need a stopwatch, a metronome, a bench or gymnasium bleacher 16¼ inches high, three chairs, and a partner to perform the test.

The exercises conducted for this test are bench-jumps, chair-dips (men) or modified push-ups (women), and bent-leg curl-ups. All exercises should be conducted with the aid of a partner. The correct procedures for performing each exercise are as follows:

■ BENCH-JUMPS

Using a bench or gymnasium bleacher 16¼ inches high, attempt to jump up and down the bench as many times as possible in a one-minute period (see Figure 2.1). If you cannot jump the full minute, you may step up and down. A repetition is counted each time both feet return to the floor.

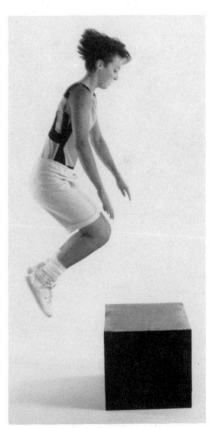

FIGURE 2.1. Bench-Jumps

■ CHAIR-DIPS

This upper-body exercise is performed by men only. Using three sturdy chairs, place one hand each on a chair, with the fingers pointing forward. Place the feet on a third chair in front of you. The hips should be bent at approximately 90 degrees. Lower your body by flexing the elbows until you reach a 90-degree angle at this joint, and then return to the starting position (see Figure 2.2). The repetition does not count if you fail to reach 90 degrees. The repetitions are performed to a two-step cadence (down-up), regulated with a metronome set at 56 beats per minute. Perform as many continuous repetitions as possible. You can no longer count the repetitions if you fail to follow the metronome cadence.

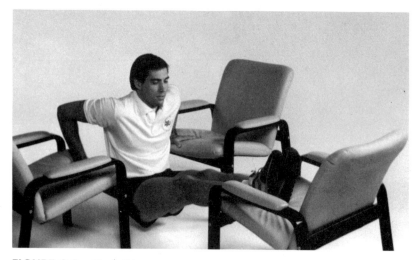

FIGURE 2.2. Chair-Dips

■ MODIFIED PUSH-UPS

Women will perform the modified push-up exercise instead of the chair-dip exercise. Lie down on the floor (face down), bend the knees (feet up in the air), and place the hands on the floor by the shoulders with the fingers pointing forward. The lower body will be supported at the knees (as opposed to the feet) throughout the test (see Figure 2.3). The chest must touch the floor on each repetition. As with the chair-dip exercise, the repetitions are performed to a two-step cadence (up-down) regulated with a metronome set at 56 beats per minute. Perform as many continuous repetitions as possible. You cannot count any more repetitions if you fail to follow the metronome cadence.

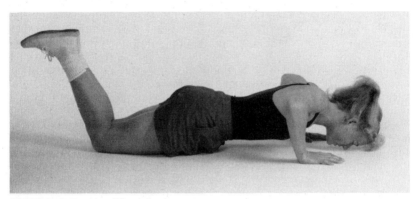

FIGURE 2.3. Modified Push-ups

■ BENT-LEG CURL-UPS

Lie down on the floor (face up) and bend both legs at the knees at approximately 100 degrees. Feet should be on the floor and you must hold them in place yourself throughout the test. Cross the arms in front of your chest, each hand on the opposite shoulder. Now raise the head off the floor, placing the chin against your chest. This is the starting and finishing position for each curl-up (see Figure 2.4a). **The back of the head may not come in contact with the floor, the hands cannot be removed from the shoulders, nor may the feet or hips be raised off the floor at any time during the test. The test is terminated if any of these four conditions occur.** When you curl up, the upper body must come to an upright position before going back down (see Figure 2.4b). The repetitions are performed to a two-step cadence (up-down) regulated with the metronome set at 40 beats per minute.

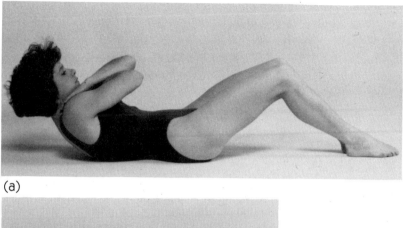

(a)

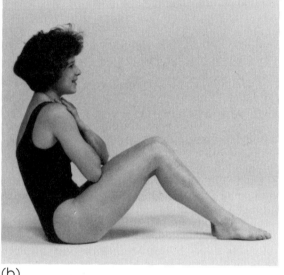

FIGURE 2.4.
Bent-Leg Curl-Ups:
starting position (a)
upright position
(b)

(b)

For this exercise, you should allow a brief practice period of five to ten seconds to familiarize yourself with the cadence (the up movement is initiated with the first beat, then you must wait for the next beat to initiate the down movement — one repetition is accomplished every two beats of the metronome). Count as many repetitions as you are able to perform following the proper cadence. The test is also terminated if you fail to maintain the appropriate cadence or if you accomplish 100 repetitions. Have your partner check the angle at the knees throughout the test to make sure that the 100-degree angle is maintained as close as possible.

According to your results, look up your percentile rank for each exercise in the far left column of Table 2.3. Next, total the percentile scores obtained for each exercise, and divide by three to obtain an average score. You can determine your individual and overall muscular endurance fitness categories according to the ratings in Table 2.4.

TABLE 2.3. Muscular Endurance Scoring Table*

MEN			
Percentile Rank	Bench Jumps	Chair Dips	Bent-leg Curl-ups
99	66	54	100
95	63	50	81
90	62	38	65
80	58	32	51
70	57	30	44
60	56	27	31
50	54	26	28
40	51	23	25
30	48	20	22
20	47	17	17
10	40	11	10
5	34	7	3
WOMEN			
Percentile Rank	Bench Jumps	Modified Push-ups	Bent-leg Curl-ups
99	58	95	100+
95	54	70	100
90	52	50	97
80	48	41	77
70	44	38	57
60	42	33	45
50	39	30	37
40	38	28	28
30	36	25	22
20	32	21	17
10	28	18	9
5	26	15	4

*Shaded area indicates recommended health-fitness standard

TABLE 2.4. Fitness Categories Based on Percentile Ranks

Average Score	Endurance Classification
80+	Excellent
60-79	Good*
40-59	Average
20-39	Fair
<19	Poor

*Recommended health-fitness standard

▬ FLEXIBILITY ASSESSMENT

Flexibility is defined as the ability of a joint to move freely through its full range of motion. The amount of muscular flexibility possessed by individuals is limited by factors such as joint structure, ligaments, tendons, muscles, skin, tissue injury, adipose tissue, body temperature, age, gender, and index of physical activity.

The development and maintenance of some level of flexibility are important components of everyone's health enhancement program — and even more so during the aging process.

Sports medicine specialists have indicated that many muscular/skeletal problems and injuries, especially among adults, are related to a lack of flexibility. Most experts agree that participating in a regular flexibility program will help a person maintain good joint mobility, increase resistance to muscle injury and soreness, prevent low back and other spinal column problems, improve and maintain good postural alignment, enhance proper and graceful body movement, improve personal appearance, improve self-image, and facilitate the development and maintenance of motor skills throughout life. Flexibility exercises have also been used successfully in the treatment of patients suffering from dysmenorrhea and general neuromuscular tension.

Stretching exercises in conjunction with calisthenics are also helpful in warm-up routines to prepare the human body for more vigorous aerobic or strength-training exercises, as well as subsequent cool-down routines to help the organism return to the normal resting state.

Two flexibility tests will be used to determine your flexibility profile. These tests are the modified sit-and-reach and the total body rotation tests.

■ MODIFIED SIT-AND-REACH TEST

To perform this test you will need the Acuflex I* sit-and-reach flexibility tester or you may simply place a yardstick on top of a box approximately 12 inches high. The procedures to administer this test are as follows:

1. Be sure to properly warm up prior to the first trial.

2. Remove your shoes for the test. Sit on the floor with your hips, back, and head against a wall, legs fully extended, and the bottom of your feet against the Acuflex I or the sit-and-reach box.

3. Place your hands one on top of the other and reach forward as far as possible without letting the hips, back, or head come off the wall. Another person should then slide the reach indicator on the Acuflex I (or yardstick) along the top of the box until the end of the indicator touches the tips of your fingers (see Figure 2.5). The indicator must then be held firmly in place throughout the rest of the test.

4. Your head and back can now come off the wall and you may gradually reach forward three times, the third time stretching forward as far as possible on the indicator (or yardstick), holding the final position for at least two seconds (see Figure 2.6). Be sure that during the test the back of the knees are kept flat against the floor. Record the final number of inches reached to the nearest one-half inch.

5. You are allowed two trials and an average of the two scores is used as the final test score. The percentile ranks and fitness categories for this test are given in Tables 2.5 and 2.4 respectively.

---

*The Acuflex I and II flexibility testers for the modified sit-and-reach and the total body rotation test can be obtained from Novel Products Figure Finder Collection, 80 Fairbanks, Unit 12, Addison, IL 60101 — (312) 628-1787.

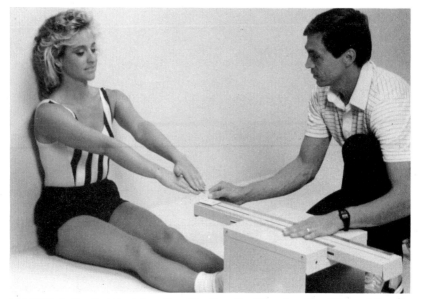

FIGURE 2.5. Determining the Starting Position for the Sit-and-Reach Test.

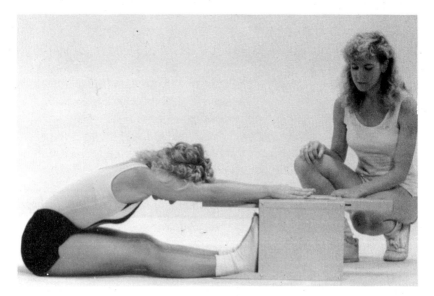

FIGURE 2.6. The Sit-and-Reach Test.

TABLE 2.5.

Percentile Ranks for the Modified Sit-and-Reach Test*

	Percentile Rank	Age Category		
		<35	36–49	50>
Men	99	24.7	18.9	16.2
	95	19.5	18.2	15.8
	90	17.9	16.1	15.0
	80	17.0	14.6	13.3
	70	15.8	13.9	12.3
	60	15.0	13.4	11.5
	50	14.4	12.6	10.2
	40	13.5	11.6	9.7
	30	13.0	10.8	9.3
	20	11.6	9.9	8.8
	10	9.2	8.3	7.8
	05	7.9	7.0	7.2
	01	7.0	5.1	4.0
Women	99	19.8	19.8	17.2
	95	18.7	19.2	15.7
	90	17.9	17.4	15.0
	80	16.7	16.2	14.2
	70	16.2	15.2	13.6
	60	15.8	14.5	12.3
	50	14.8	13.5	11.1
	40	14.5	12.8	10.1
	30	13.7	12.2	9.2
	20	12.6	11.0	8.3
	10	10.1	9.7	7.5
	05	8.1	8.5	3.7
	01	2.6	2.0	1.5

*Shaded area indicates recommended health-fitness standard

■ TOTAL BODY ROTATION TEST

An Acuflex II total body rotation flexibility tester or a measuring scale with a sliding panel is needed to administer this test. The Acuflex II or scale is placed on the wall at shoulder height and should be adjustable to accommodate individual differences in height. If you need to build your own scale, use two measuring tapes and glue them above and below the sliding panel — centered at the 15-inch mark. Each tape should be at least 30 inches long. If no sliding panel is available, simply tape the measuring tapes onto a wall. A line must also be drawn on the floor which is centered with the 15-inch mark (see Figures 2.7, 2.8, 2.9, and 2.10). The following procedures should be used for this test:

1. Be sure to properly warm up prior to initiating this test.

2. To start, you should stand sideways, an arm's length away from the wall, with the feet straight ahead, slightly separated, and the toes right up to the corresponding line drawn on the floor. The arm opposite to the wall is held out horizontally from the body, making a fist with the hand. The Acuflex II, measuring scale, or tapes should be shoulder height at this time.

3. You can now rotate the body, the extended arm going backward (always maintaining a horizontal plane) and making contact with the panel, gradually sliding it forward as far as possible. If no panel is available, slide the fist alongside the tapes as far as possible. The final position must be held for at least two seconds. The hand should be positioned with the little finger side forward during the entire sliding movement, as illustrated in Figure 2.11. **It is crucial that the proper hand position be used. Many people will attempt to either open the hand, push with extended fingers, or slide the panel with the knuckles; none of which is an acceptable test procedure. During the test, the knees can be slightly bent, but the feet cannot be moved, always pointing straight forward.** The body must be kept as straight (vertical) as possible.

4. The test is conducted on either the right or left side of the body. You are allowed two trials on each side. The farthest point reached, measured to the nearest one-half inch, and held for at least two seconds is recorded. The average of the

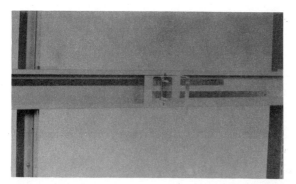

FIGURE 2.7.
Acuflex II Measuring Device for the Total Body Rotation Test.

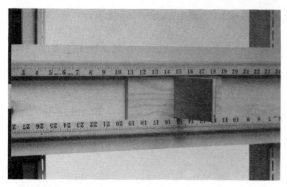

FIGURE 2.8.
Homemade Measuring Device for the Total Body Rotation Test.

FIGURE 2.9.
Measuring Tapes for the Total Body Rotation Test.

two trials is used as the final test score. Using Tables 2.6 and 2.4, you can determine the respective percentile rank and flexibility fitness classification for this test.

After obtaining your score and percentile rank for both tests, you can determine the overall flexibility fitness classification by computing an average percentile rank from the two tests and using the same guidelines given in Table 2.4.

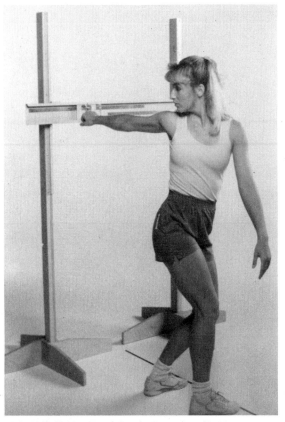

FIGURE 2.10. Total Body Rotation Test.

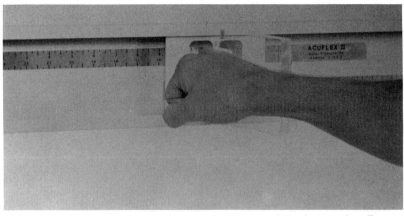

FIGURE 2.11. Proper Hand Position for the Total Body Rotation Test.

TABLE 2.6.

Percentile Ranks for the Total Body Rotation Test

	Percentile Rank	Age:	Right Rotation <35	36–49	50>	Left Rotation <35	36–49	50>
	99		27.8	25.2	22.2	28.0	26.6	21.0
	95		25.6	23.8	20.7	24.8	24.5	20.0
	90		24.1	22.5	19.3	23.6	23.0	17.7
	80		22.3	21.0	16.3	22.0	21.2	15.5
	70		20.7	18.7	15.7	20.3	20.4	14.7
	60		19.0	17.3	14.7	19.3	18.7	13.9
Men	50		17.2	16.3	12.3	18.0	16.7	12.7
	40		16.3	14.7	11.5	16.8	15.3	11.7
	30		15.0	13.3	10.7	15.0	14.8	10.3
	20		13.3	11.2	8.7	13.3	13.7	9.5
	10		11.3	8.0	2.7	10.5	10.8	4.3
	05		8.3	5.5	0.3	8.9	8.8	0.3
	01		2.9	2.0	0.0	1.7	5.1	0.0
	99		29.4	27.1	21.7	28.6	27.1	23.0
	95		25.3	25.9	19.7	24.8	25.3	21.4
	90		23.0	21.3	19.0	23.0	23.4	20.5
	80		20.8	19.6	17.9	21.5	20.2	19.1
	70		19.3	17.3	16.8	20.5	18.6	17.3
	60		18.0	16.5	15.6	19.3	17.7	16.0
Women	50		17.3	14.6	14.0	18.0	16.4	14.8
	40		16.0	13.1	12.8	17.2	14.8	13.7
	30		15.2	11.7	8.5	15.7	13.6	10.0
	20		14.0	9.8	3.9	15.2	11.6	6.3
	10		11.1	6.1	2.2	13.6	8.5	3.0
	05		8.8	4.0	1.1	7.3	6.8	0.7
	01		3.2	2.8	0.0	5.3	4.3	0.0

Reproduced with permission from Hoeger, W. W. K. *Lifetime Physican Fitness & Wellness: A Personalized Program.* Morton Publishing Company, 1989.

BODY COMPOSITION

The term "body composition" is used in reference to the fat and nonfat components of the human body. The fat component is usually referred to as fat mass or percent body fat. The nonfat component is referred to as lean body mass. Although for many years people have relied on height/weight charts to determine ideal body weight, we now know that these tables can be highly inaccurate for many people. The proper way of determining ideal weight is through body composition, that is, by finding out what percent of total body weight is fat and what amount is lean tissue. Once the fat percentage is known, ideal body weight can be calculated from ideal body fat or the recommended amount where there is no detriment to human health.

The importance of ideal body composition in the achievement and maintenance of good health can not be underestimated. Obesity has become a health hazard of epidemic proportions in most developed countries around the world. Obesity by itself has been associated with several serious health problems and accounts for 15 to 20 percent of the annual U.S. mortality rate. Obesity has long been recognized as a major risk factor for diseases of the cardiovascular system, including coronary heart disease, hypertension, congestive heart failure, elevated blood lipids, atherosclerosis, strokes, thromboembolitic disease, varicose veins, and intermittent claudication.

In spite of the fact that different techniques used to determine percent body fat were developed several years ago, many people are still unaware of these procedures and continue to depend on height/weight charts to find out what their "ideal" body weight should be. These standard height/weight tables were first published in 1912 and were based on average weights (including shoes and clothing) for men and women who obtained life insurance policies between 1888 and 1905. The ideal weight on the tables is obtained according to sex, height, and frame size. Since no scientific guidelines to determine frame size are given, most people choose their size based on the column where their body weight is found.

To determine whether people are truly obese or "falsely" at ideal body weight, body composition must be established. Obesity is related to excessive body fat accumulation. If body weight is used as the only criteria, an individual can easily be overweight according to height/weight charts, and yet not be obese. This is commonly seen among football players, body builders, weight lifters, and other athletes with large muscle size. Some of these athletes in reality have very little body fat and appear to be twenty or thirty pounds overweight.

On the other end of the spectrum, some people who weigh very little and are viewed by many as "skinny" or underweight can actually be classified as obese because of their high body fat content. Not at all uncommon are cases of people weighing as little as 100 pounds who are over 30 percent fat (about one-third of their total body weight). Such cases are more readily observed among sedentary people and those who are constantly dieting. Both physical inactivity and constant negative caloric balance lead to a loss in lean body mass. It is clear from these examples that body weight alone does not always tell the true story.

Total fat in the human body is classified into two types, essential fat and storage fat. The essential fat is needed for normal physiological functions, and without it, human health begins to deteriorate. This essential fat constitutes about 3 percent of the total fat in men and 12 percent in women. The percentage is higher in women because it includes sex-specific fat, such as found in the breast tissue, the uterus, and other sex-related fat deposits. Storage fat constitutes the fat that is stored in adipose tissue, mostly beneath the skin (subcutaneous fat) and around major organs in the body.

The assessment of body composition is most frequently done using skinfold thickness. This technique is based on the principle that approximately 50 percent of the fatty tissue in the body is deposited directly beneath the skin. If this tissue is estimated validly and reliably, a good indication of percent body fat can be obtained. This test is regularly performed with the aid of pressure calipers (see Figure 2.12), and several sites must be measured to reflect the total percentage of fat. These sites are triceps, suprailium, and

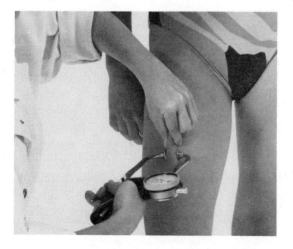

FIGURE 2.12.
Skinfold Thickness Technique for Body Composition Assessment

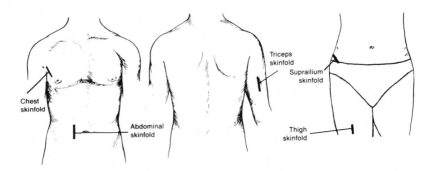

FIGURE 2.13. Anatomical Landmarks for Skinfolds

thigh skinfolds for women; and chest, abdomen, and thigh for men (see Figure 2.13). All measurements should be taken on the right side of the body with the subject standing. The correct anatomical landmarks for skinfolds are:

Chest: a diagonal fold halfway between the shoulder crease and the nipple.

Abdomen: a vertical fold about one inch to the right of the umbilicus.

Triceps: a vertical fold on the back of the upper arm, half-way between the shoulder and the arm.

Thigh: a diagonal fold on the front of the thigh, mid-way between the knee and the hip.

Suprailium: a diagonal fold above the crest of the ilium (on the side of the hip).

Each site is measured by grasping a double thickness of skin firmly with the thumb and forefinger, pulling the fold slightly away from the muscle tissue. Hold the calipers perpendicular to the fold, and take the measurements one-half inch below the finger hold. Measure each site three times and read the values to the nearest .1 to .5 mm. Record the average of the two closest readings as the final value. Take the readings without delay to avoid excessive compression of the skinfold. Releasing and refolding the skinfold is required between readings. After determining the average value for each site you can determine your percent fat using the nomogram given in Figure 2.14. The recommended percent body fat based on age and gender is given in Table 2.7. You may also compute your recommended body weight using the computation form given in Figure 2.15.

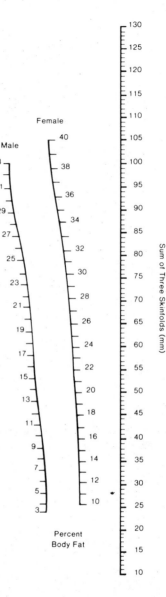

From "A nomogram for the estimate of percent body fat from generalized equations" by W. B. Baun, M. R. Baun, and P. B. Raven, Research Quarterly for Exercise and Sport, vol. 52, 1981, pp. 380-384. Reprinted by permission.

FIGURE 2.14. Nomogram for percent fat determination from the sum of three skinfold sites. The sites for men are the chest, abdomen, and thigh. For women, the sites are the triceps, thigh, and suprailium. Based on age and the sum of the three skinfolds, place a ruler over the nomogram and find the percent body fat in the respective gender column.

TABLE 2.7.

Recommended Body Composition According to Percent Body Fat

Age	Males	Females
<29	12-20%	17-25%
30-49	13-21%	18-26%
50>	14-22%	19-27%

A. Current Body Weight (BW): _____ lbs

B. Current Percent Fat (%F)*: _____%

C. Fat Weight (FW) = BW × %F = _____ × _____ = lbs

D. Lean Body Mass (LBM) = BW − FW = _____ − _____ = lbs

E. Age: _____

F. Recommended Fat Percent (RFP — see Table 2.7): _____ %

G. Recommended Body Weight (RBW) = LBM/(1.0 − RFP)

   RBW = _____ / (1.0 − _____) = _____ lbs

*Express percentages in decimal form (e.g., 25% = .25)

FIGURE 2.15. Recommended Body Weight Determination

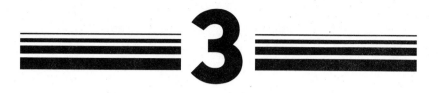

Water Aerobics Fitness Program

Water aerobics provides fitness, fun, and safety for people of all ages. The popularity of aquatic exercise has grown from an initial 200,000 participants in 1983 to approximately 2.5 million in 1989. Water aerobics is a major reason for this dramatic increase and consequently it has become one of the fastest growing fitness activities in the United States. According to most experts, this trend will continue to increase by leaps and bounds over the next decade.

Water aerobics contributes to overall fitness development by providing increased resistance (water) with virtually no impact to the participant. This relatively "new" fitness activity has become the perfect alternative to traditional land-based programs that are contraindicated for people with muscular-skeletal problems. Furthermore, most land-based activities place such a tremendous amount of stress on the human body that over half of all new participants drop out within the first six weeks due to injuries. Participants of all ages and both genders are finding out that fitness, the water aerobics way, is fun, without the pain and agony of injuries.

This chapter will address the implementation of a complete water aerobics fitness program. The basic principles of water exercise, injury prevention, the water aerobics class, a large variety of water exercises, and a sample class sequence are discussed in detail to help you obtain the full benefits of your water aerobics program.

BASIC PRINCIPLES OF WATER EXERCISE

Due to the greater density of water, the aquatic environment is a different exercise medium than air. Land-based activities rely on gravity to provide the necessary overload for fitness development. In the aquatic environment, the overload is primarily accomplished through the resistance provided by the water. It is important, however, to learn how to use the water to develop optimal resistance.

Hydrodynamic Principles

Application of the overload principle is the fundamental concept required for improvements in the various systems of the body. This principle states that to improve the condition of the body, the demands placed on the various systems must be greater than those to which they are normally accustomed. This overload, gradually intensified over a period of time, causes the various systems of the body to adjust and increase their capacity to do work.

During water aerobics, the overload to develop cardiovascular endurance, muscle tone (strength and endurance), and flexibility is created by the added resistance provided by the water. Hydrodynamic principles, however, affect how the body moves through water and are essential for a discussion on how to develop resistance.

The most important of the hydrodynamic principles is the drag force or increased resistance that is created by the density of water. Due to the drag force, movements such as walking in water require a greater effort than on land. This added resistance is the key stimulus for cardiovascular and strength development.

In aquatic exercises, the speed of limb movement (also a hydrodynamic principle) is directly proportional to the force applied to the respective limb. Due to the drag force of water, resistance increases rapidly as the speed of movement increases. This concept is significant during water aerobics. The speed at which the arms and legs are moved through the water must be fast enough to provide sufficient resistance for cardiovascular development, that is, to elevate the heart rate to an optimal training zone. Your optimal training zone or target training zone is discussed under The Water Aerobics Class section in this chapter.

Speed of movement is also important during toning exercises. The speed of an exercise has to be of sufficient magnitude to generate the necessary overload for muscular development. To feel the effect of the speed of movement and the drag force, try a slow biceps curl in water, followed by a fast curl. A greater resistance is encountered during the fast curl.

Another hydrodynamic principle relates to the length of the exercising limb (lever). As the length of a lever increases, a greater force is required to overcome the resistance. Conversely, a shorter lever requires less of an effort to overcome the resistance. This principle is especially important during the aerobic phase of the exercise session. The more muscle force required, the greater the demand on the cardiovascular system. This is also important when modifying your exercises. If you are training above your target heart rate zone, you can reduce your workload by simply shortening the exercising lever. Lengthening the lever will increase the workload. An example of this law can be experienced by flexing the elbow as opposed to flexing (raising) the entire arm under water. Flexing the elbow requires less effort than flexing the entire arm. Please note that to prevent injuries when using long levers (e.g., moving the entire arm), joints should be kept "soft" and not locked.

A final hydrodynamic principle relates primarily to the hand position in the water. As the surface area increases, so does the amount of resistance necessary to move the body (or selected body part). It requires less energy to move a fist through the water than a hand that is held in a slightly cupped position (see Figure 3.1). This is a significant principle when modifying exercise intensity. If you find that you are working too hard, closing the hand will reduce some of the water resistance. Try this exercise yourself by moving your hand in a fist and a slightly cupped position under the water. You should be able to feel the difference between the forces required to move the hand in these two positions.

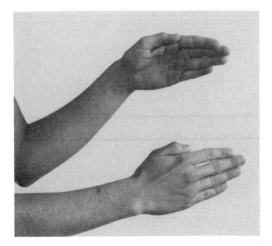

FIGURE 3.1. Paddle or cupped hand position used during most water aerobic exercises.

Special Considerations for Water Aerobics

■ WATER DEPTH

The depth of the water will determine the amount of resistance that you encounter as well as the impact that the joints receive during your workout. The recommended depth for all standing water exercises ranges from two to three inches above the umbilicus (navel) to armpit level (see Figure 3.2). If you exercise in shallower water, the buoyancy effect is reduced; consequently, your body will weigh more and the impact on joints and tendons will be greater. On the other hand, if you exercise in water deeper than recommended, your body will become so buoyant that it will be difficult to create sufficient resistance to elevate the heart rate. You will need to try different water depths, within the recommended range, to find your optimal training depth.

■ POOL SURFACE

The bottom surface of the pool should be smooth and reasonably flat. Most pools slope gradually to greater depths, which will provide a variety of exercising levels that you can choose from. Do not, however, attempt to exercise on steep slopes because injuries or slipping could occur.

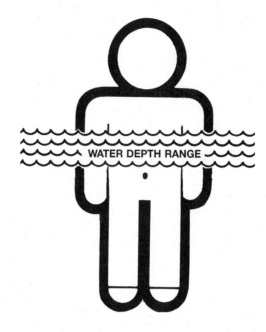

FIGURE 3.2. Water depth for standing aerobic exercises should range from two to three inches above the umbilicus to armpit level.

■ **CONTACT WITH THE BOTTOM OF THE POOL**

All aquatic exercises can be performed with bare feet. The buoyancy provided by the water renders a cushioning effect that eliminates the need of foot protection for most people. Proper landing, however, is still important. When contacting the bottom of the pool, land on the ball of the foot and roll the foot downward toward the heel (never land on your heel).

■ **WATER TEMPERATURE**

The most comfortable temperature range for water aerobics ranges from 78 to 84 degrees Fahrenheit. If the pool temperature is colder, you will need to warm up for a longer period of time and you will probably want to conduct your flexibility exercises after the aerobic phase instead of at the end of the class. Pool temperatures warmer than 86-88 degrees Fahrenheit can be hazardous during exercise. Muscles produce heat during exercise. If the water temperature is too high, the combination of warm water and increased body heat may lead to heat exhaustion or even heat stroke. Untreated heat stroke can be fatal.

■ ARMS IN VS ARMS OUT

Because of the hydrodynamic principles, greater resistances can be developed by exercising with arms in the water as opposed to outside the water. Is it ever appropriate, however, to exercise with the arms out of the water? There is some controversy regarding this issue. Some instructors feel that when the arms are out of the water it is difficult to elevate the heart rate to obtain adequate training benefits. They also feel that lack of arm control can cause back strain and lead to potential back injury. In the opinion of the authors of this book, arm exercises out of the water are appropriate if such movements are controlled or restricted within safe limits of the joints' range of motion. The use of these exercises should also be limited to short periods of time and combined with strong leg actions. Such practice will still maintain the heart rate in the optimal training zone. It will also allow you to work the shoulder muscles through their entire range of motion. Additionally, intermittent arm movements out of the water provide variety to your workout. If at any time you are uncomfortable with the arm position, modify the exercise by lowering the arms or eliminate the action entirely.

■ MUSIC

Your instructor may or may not use music during the water aerobics class. The acoustics of most pools are not suitable for you to be able to listen to the instructor and the music at the same time. Also, keep in mind that electrical wires are not allowed near water; therefore, only battery charged cassette players should be operated. If music is used, the cadence should be set at about 120 beats per minute. Faster cadences tend to promote improper exercise technique. Whether music is used or not, you will need to set a tempo that will be challenging and still allow you time to complete each exercise action.

■ SPECIAL TIPS

1. **What kind of suit should I wear?** One-piece swimsuits are recommended for comfort and mobility. For most participants, the modern tank suits will be sufficient. For those

requiring additional support for the breast, there are swim-suit styles that have shelf bras built in or a bra can actually be sewn in.

2. **Can I keep my hair dry?** Yes, it is possible to execute shallow water exercises without getting your hair wet. Water will, nonetheless, splash up occasionally. A shower hat or swimming cap will help keep your hair dry.

3. **If foot protection is needed, what should I do?** If the bottom of the pool is rough, cotton socks can be worn. Scuba diving booties can also provide foot and ankle support when such is required.

INJURY PREVENTION

Although water aerobics is much safer than land-based activities, there are inherent risks associated with any activity. There is always an assumption of risk when taking part in any exercise program. Many of the potential injuries can be minimized by taking some precautions and following a few simple guidelines.

1. *Always exercise in a supervised environment.* If you are at a lake front or a pool, a lifeguard should be present. If you have a pool in your backyard, make sure that you exercise under supervision and that you and your family understand basic water rescue methods. Contact your local Red Cross, YMCA, or YWCA for more information.

2. *Follow basic monitoring techniques.* Check your exercise intensity frequently. Always pay attention to pain and modify your exercise sessions accordingly.

3. *Keep all motions controlled in the water environment.* Place the limb as opposed to flinging it (all movements should have specific starting and finishing positions).

4. *Limit twisting actions.* Injuries are often the result of too much momentum being generated in the water through uncontrolled twisting actions.

5. *Protect your joints by keeping them soft, not locked.*

Learn to Listen to Your Body

A key principle in exercise prescription is that all programs must be individualized to meet each person's needs. You need to understand that our bodies are not all alike. Fitness levels vary among individuals. People do not respond to training in the same manner. Individuals are also prone to different types of injuries.

It is important that you learn to listen to your body. If you feel tired, you should reduce the intensity of the exercise. If you are feeling great, put more energy into the activity. Furthermore, it is conceivable that a particular exercise that feels great to most participants may cause some discomfort to you. Pain is nature's way of letting you know that something is wrong. If you experience pain or undue discomfort with a given exercise, you should discontinue the exercise and notify your instructor, who may be able to pinpoint the reason for the discomfort. There is a possibility that you are executing the exercise incorrectly or that a particular exercise is not for you. You will be able to prevent potential injuries by paying attention to pain signals and making adjustments accordingly. Modify the exercises to fit your needs.

Water Exercise and Cramps

Muscle cramps may also occur during exercise. Cramps are caused by the body's depletion of essential electrolytes, a breakdown in the coordination between opposing muscle groups, or a decrease in blood flow to active muscle tissue due to tight clothing. If you have a muscle cramp, initially you should attempt to stretch the muscles involved. For example, in the case of the calf muscle, pull your toes up toward the knees. After stretching the muscle, do some mild exercises that require the use of that particular muscle.

In many instances, and primarily in pregnant and lactating women, muscle cramps are related to a lack of calcium. Women who experience cramps during these periods are given calcium supplements, which usually relieves the problem.

Water Aerobics and Pregnancy

There is no reason why women should not exercise during pregnancy. If anything, it is desirable that women do so to strengthen the body and prepare for delivery. Physically fit women experience easier delivery and faster recovery as compared to unfit women. The final decision for exercise participation, nevertheless, should be made between the woman and her personal physician.

Experts have recommended that a woman who has been exercising regularly may continue to carry out the same activity through the fifth month of pregnancy, but care should be taken not to exceed a working heart rate of 140 beats per minute. After the fifth month, walking, stationary cycling, moderate swimming, and/or modified water aerobic exercises are indicated in conjunction with some light strengthening exercises. For women that have not exercised regularly, twenty to thirty minutes of daily walking and light strengthening exercises are recommended throughout the entire pregnancy.

THE WATER AEROBICS CLASS

The main purpose of the water aerobics class is to develop overall physical fitness. To meet this goal safely and effectively, your workout or water aerobics class will be broken down into four phases: warm-up, aerobic, toning (strength and endurance development), and flexibility. Each of these phases will be discussed in detail.

Setting Realistic Fitness Goals

Before discussing the four phases of the water aerobics class, it is imperative that you consider your fitness goals. Your goals will help you determine your attitude toward the entire program. In our modern world we have become accustomed to "quick fixes" with everything from fast food to one-hour dry cleaning. There is, however, no "quick fix" for fitness. Fitness takes time and dedication to develop. In the end, however, the benefits of a better quality of life will be well worth your effort. By determining realistic fitness goals you can get a better view of the overall picture. Progress and improvements can be charted which will help you adhere to your fitness commitment. Figure 3.3 contains a goal-setting chart that will help you determine your goals. You are encouraged to take the time now to sit down and fill it out.

Indicate below two or three general goals that you will work on during the next few weeks and write the specific objectives that you will use to accomplish each goal (you may not need five specific objectives, only write as many as you need).

General Goal: _____

Specific Objectives:

1. _____

2. _____

3. _____

4. _____

5. _____

General Goal: _____

Specific Objectives:

1. _____

2. _____

3. _____

4. _____

5. _____

General Goal: _____

Specific Objectives:

1. _____

2. _____

3. _____

4. _____

5. _____

FIGURE 3.3. Goal Setting Chart

Warm-up Phase

The purpose of the warm-up is to prepare the body for exercise. The warm-up is important because it prepares you for the aerobic phase and helps lower the risk of injuries. The warm-up achieves its purpose by gradually increasing blood flow to the exercising muscles, elevating internal body temperature to the point of mild perspiration (by about one degree Fahrenheit), and increasing joint range of motion. Under normal conditions, this phase lasts five to ten minutes. If the temperature of the air and/or water is lower than recommended, warm-up time should be extended by another five to seven minutes. During this phase, all initial joint movements should be executed slowly and gradually, progressing from a small range of motion to a full range of motion.

The warm-up can be segmented into three parts: (a) isolation exercises or those that help create body awareness (i.e., working one body part at a time, such as knee lifts); (b) actual warm-up exercises, which usually involve large muscle groups and mirror at a slower pace the exercises that will follow in the aerobic phase; and (c) pre-stretches or flexibility exercises, which are executed only after the internal body temperature has been elevated (increased body temperature improves the effectiveness of flexibility exercises). The muscles that should be pre-stretched are those that will have the greatest stress placed upon them during the aerobic phase. Pre-stretching these muscle groups will make them more pliable and less prone to injury. Each stretch should be held a minimum of 10 seconds, but preferably 30 seconds.

Aerobic Phase

The objective of the aerobic phase is to improve the capacity of the cardiovascular system. To accomplish this development, the heart muscle has to be overloaded like any other muscle in the human body. There are four basic principles that govern the development of this system. These principles are intensity, mode, duration, and frequency of exercise.

1. **Intensity of Exercise.** This principle refers to how hard a person has to exercise to improve cardiovascular endurance. This is accomplished by increasing the heart rate to a target training zone or target heart rate zone. The stimuli

is provided by making the heart pump at a rate between 60 and 80 percent of the heart's reserve capacity. These two percentages are easily calculated and training can be monitored by checking your pulse. The following steps are used to determine the intensity of exercise or target training zone.

A. Estimate your maximal heart rate (Max. HR). This is done using the following formula:

Max. HR = 210* minus age (210 − age)

B. Take your resting heart rate (RHR). This is done by counting your pulse on the wrist by placing two or three fingers over the radial artery (forearm on the side of the thumb) or over the carotid artery in the neck just below the jaw next to your voice box. Count your pulse for one full minute to obtain your resting heart rate. Always start your count with zero.

C. Determine the heart rate reserve (HRR). This is accomplished by subtracting the RHR from the maximal heart rate (HRR = Max. HR − RHR).

D. The target training zone is determined by computing the training intensities (TI) at 60 and 80 percent. Multiply the heart rate reserve by the respective 60 and 80 percentages and then add the resting heart rate to both of these figures (60 percent TI = HRR × .60 + RHR, and 80 percent TI = HRR × .80 + RHR). Your target training zone is found between these two target heart rates. For safety and conditioning purposes, it is recommended that beginners train at the 60 percent level during the first six to eight weeks of exercise. Following this initial conditioning period, they may move up closer to the 80 percent level.

---

*210 is used for aquatic exercise (as opposed to 220 on land) because research indicates that maximal heart rates in water are approximately 10 beats per minute lower than on land.

E. *Example.* The cardiovascular training zone in water for a 20-year-old person with a resting heart rate of 72 bpm would be:

Max. HR: 210 − 20 = 190 bpm
RHR = 72 bpm
HRR: 190 − 72 = 118 beats
60 Percent TI = (118 × .60) + 72 = 143 bpm
80 Percent TI = (118 × .80) + 72 = 166 bpm
Target training zone: 143 to 166 bpm

The target training zone indicates that whenever you exercise to improve the cardiovascular system, you have to maintain the heart rate between the 60 and 80 percent training intensities to obtain adequate development. After a few weeks of training, you should experience a significant reduction in resting heart rate (10 to 20 beats in 8 to 12 weeks); therefore, you should recompute your target zone periodically.

2. **Mode of Exercise.** The type of exercise that develops the cardiovascular system has to be aerobic in nature. Once you have established your cardiovascular training zone, any activity or combination of activities that will get your heart rate up to that training zone and keep it there for as long as you exercise will yield adequate development. In addition to water aerobics, examples of such activities are walking, jogging, aerobic dancing, swimming, cross-country skiing, rope skipping, cycling, racquetball, stair climbing, and stationary running or cycling.

3. **Duration of Exercise.** It is recommended that a person maintain the heart rate in the target training zone between 15 and 60 minutes per session. The duration is based on how intensely a person trains. If the training is done around 80 percent of HRR, 15 to 20 minutes are sufficient. At 60 percent intensity, the person should train for at least 30 minutes.

4. **Frequency of Exercise.** Ideally, a person should engage in aerobic exercise four or five days per week. Research has indicated that to maintain cardiovascular fitness, a training

session should be conducted about every 48 hours. Three 20- to 30-minute training sessions per week, done on non-consecutive days, will maintain cardiovascular endurance as long as the heart rate is in the appropriate target zone.

The goal of the aerobic phase in your water aerobics workout is to elevate the heart rate to the target training zone and maintain that rate for 15-30 minutes. Beginning classes should start with 15 minutes per class session and then gradually increase the duration by about five minutes per week.

You should also realize that the aerobic phase is usually divided into three parts: (a) a gradual heart rate increase to the target zone, which lasts two to five minutes; (b) the actual aerobic workout, where the heart rate is maintained in the target zone for 15 to 30 minutes; and (c) the aerobic cool-down, where the heart rate is gradually lowered toward near resting level. It is important that you not stop abruptly following aerobic exercise. This will cause blood to pool in the exercised body parts, thereby diminishing the return of blood to the heart. A decreased blood return can cause dizziness, faintness, or even induce cardiac abnormalities.

To monitor the target training zone, you will need to know how to take your exercise heart rate. This is also done by checking your pulse on the radial or the carotid artery. Caution should be used when taking the pulse at the carotid artery because too much pressure on the artery may slow the heart and the measurement will be inaccurate. When you check the heart rate, begin with zero and count the number of beats in a ten second period, then multiply by six to get the per-minute pulse rate. Exercise heart rate should not be taken for a full minute because the heart rate begins to slow down 15 seconds following exercise cessation. Do not hesitate, however, to stop during your exercise bout to check your pulse; it is difficult to feel the pulse while exercising.

After obtaining the exercise heart rate, compare this number with the heart rate range that you calculated under intensity of exercise. Your heart rate should fall between the two numbers that you determined for your range. If the rate is too low, increase the intensity of the exercise. If the rate is too high, slow down. You may want to practice taking your pulse outside of class to become familiar with these monitoring techniques.

For the first few weeks of your water aerobics class, heart rates during the aerobic phase should be monitored every three to four minutes. As you become familiar with your body's response to exercise, you may only have to monitor the heart rate twice during the aerobic phase: once at five to seven minutes into this phase, and a second time near the end of the phase.

Another technique that is sometimes used to determine your exercise intensity is by talking during exercise and then taking the pulse immediately thereafter. Learning to associate the degree of difficulty when talking to the actual exercise heart rate will allow you to develop a sense of how hard you are working. Generally, if you can talk easily, you are not working hard enough. If you can talk but are slightly breathless, you should be close to the target range. If you cannot talk at all, you are working too hard.

Tempo Considerations

Tempo refers to the actual speed of limb movement through the water. The tempo of each exercise must be such that it will allow you to complete each action and at the same time generate an optimal amount of resistance. If during the aerobic phase the tempo is too fast, you won't be able to complete the exercise action. As a result, the tendency will be to shorten your limb (lever arm). This in turn will reduce the overload and decrease your training benefits. During the toning phase if the tempo is too fast, the tendency will be to either shorten the lever arm or limit the joint's range of the motion — defeating the purpose of the exercise. On the other hand, a slow tempo during either phase (aerobic or toning) will not provide enough resistance for adequate fitness gains. One of your challenges will be to find the correct tempo to adequately pace yourself throughout the workout.

Pacing

The concept of pacing to achieve safe and comfortable exercise limits is necessary to make your exercise session a positive experience. This is crucial because people do not enjoy participating in painful activities. Yet, all too frequently people think that exercise has to hurt to be beneficial. The "no pain, no gain" philosophy is not only untrue, but dangerous as well. Research has proven that fitness gains can be obtained by exercising within the comfortable and safe limits provided by your target heart rate range. In addition, there is a lower chance of overuse injuries by exercising within safe limits. Injuries are a major reason why so many beginners drop out of fitness programs.

Another principle that you must understand is that you don't have to keep up with the instructor or the person next to you. Your instructor is an example of what you may do, but not what you have to do at this point. It is important to remember that exercise programs must be individualized. You need to set your own pace and the only person that you need to keep up with is yourself.

Toning Phase

The purpose of the toning phase is to develop muscular strength and endurance. Adequate levels of strength and endurance are necessary for optimal performance in daily activities such as sitting, walking, running, lifting and carrying objects, doing housework, or even for the enjoyment of recreational activities. Adequate strength and endurance also help decrease the risk of injury. Furthermore, increased tone is important because even at rest muscle tissue burns more calories than fat. As you tone, you increase muscle tissue and decrease fat. This in turn raises your resting metabolic rate, which in the long run, helps in weight reduction and/or weight maintenance.

Although muscular strength and endurance are interrelated, a basic difference exists between the two. Strength is defined as the ability to exert maximum force against resistance. Endurance is the ability of a muscle to exert submaximal force repeatedly over a period of time.

Muscular strength and endurance development are accomplished through the overload principle. Based on the previous definitions, muscular strength is developed through exercises that require muscle contraction against a large resistance. Consequently, only a few repetitions can be performed (less than 10 repetitions maximum). Muscular endurance is developed by performing exercises against a smaller resistance; henceforth, many repetitions can be performed.

In water aerobics, the nature of the environment is more conducive to endurance exercises. This is fine, because life's daily activities require mostly muscular endurance as opposed to strength. In this regard, toning exercises will be done in sets (or series) of many repetitions such as 3 sets of 15 repetitions.

When performing the toning exercises you should feel as though the muscle is working hard, but you don't necessarily have to "go for the burn." Execute the number of repetitions that you are capable of doing, and when you start feeling uncomfortable, try one more and then stop. After your muscles have had a short rest interval, start the next set. As the days progress, try to increase the number of repetitions that you can do. You may wish to write the number of repetitions down after each class to view your overall progress. Due to time constraints, it is recommended that upper body exercises be emphasized one day and lower body exercises the next.

During the toning phase, it is important to breathe as normally as possible. If you hold your breath during each repetition, an effect called the valsalva maneuver may cause high intercostal blood pressure, which may be dangerous for some individuals.

Special Equipment for Toning Exercises

There are many types of specialized equipment on the market today that can be purchased for use in water aerobics. Inexpensive equipment, however, can be used to enhance the toning exercises. The purpose of this equipment is either to provide a more effective exercise position, as in the case of the milk jugs (which allows you to work both legs simultaneously), or to place a greater overload on the exercising muscles, such as when using hand paddles or the pull buoy. The equipment items that are discussed next are only those that are available at most swimming pools or can be easily obtained.

■ HAND PADDLES

Swimmers have used hand paddles for a long time to increase the surface area and the resistance that can be developed in the water. Hand paddles can be used for the same purpose in your water aerobic class, as shown in Figure 3.4.

Extra precautions are needed when using paddles. The increased resistance and surface area that are created when paddles are used allow the participant to generate greater momentum, which could cause injury if not properly controlled. Furthermore,

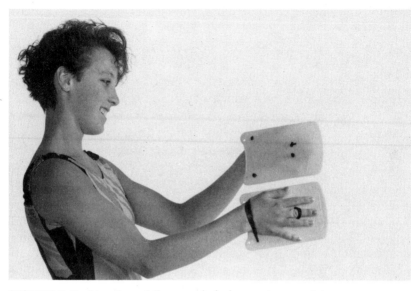

FIGURE 3.4. Hand paddles used during water aerobics.

stopping or slowing the action requires greater muscular force. To protect the joints when using the paddles follow these simple guidelines:

1. Begin each exercise with a slow motion until you get used to the hand paddles.
2. Do not fully extend the limbs (keep the joints soft).
3. Keep all arm actions under control.
4. Use hand paddles only during the toning phase.
5. Hand paddles are recommended for toning exercises 45, 46, 47, 48, 49, 51, 52, 54 and 55 at the end of this chapter.

■ PULL BUOYS

Swimmers frequently use pull buoys to keep the legs afloat. During toning exercises, buoyancy provided by the pull buoy can be used to provide more resistance for the thigh and buttock muscles. Extra care should be taken when putting on the pull buoy. To do so, loosen the strap and slide your foot between the two floats. Now, tighten the strap sufficiently to hold the pull buoy in place, but keep it loose enough for comfort (see Figure 3.5).

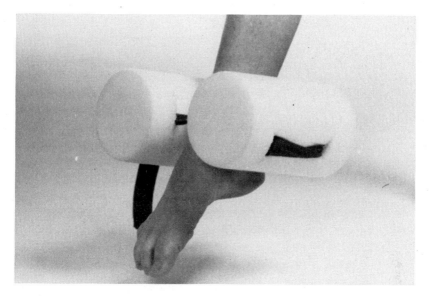

FIGURE 3.5. Pull buoys are frequently used during toning exercises in water aerobics.

The following guidelines are recommended when using the pull buoy:

1. Use the pull buoy on one foot at a time only.
2. Sit on the side of the pool or brace yourself adequately when putting on the pull buoy.
3. The pull buoy should be used only while holding onto the side of the pool.
4. Keep the exercise tempo slow and controlled at all times.
5. Use the pull buoy only during the toning phase.
6. Pull buoys are recommended for use with exercises: 57, 58 and 59 at the end of this chapter.

■ MILK JUGS

One-gallon milk jug containers (with lids) can be used as flotation devices to provide a more effective exercise position for the legs and the buttock area. Exercising with milk jugs requires a pool depth of at least four feet; therefore, these exercises are limited to individuals who are comfortable in deep water. Lifeguard supervision is mandatory.

To use the milk jugs, grasp the handles and place the jugs beneath your arms as shown in Figure 3.6. Your feet should be clear of the pool bottom as you float in the vertical position. Exercises 65 to 71 at the end of this chapter are for use with milk jugs.

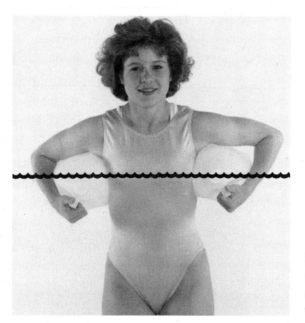

FIGURE 3.6. Use of milk jugs during a water aerobics workout.

Flexibility

The purpose of this phase in water aerobics is to increase the range of motion of the joints. Regular flexibility exercises will help a person maintain good joint mobility, increase resistance to muscle injury and soreness, prevent low back and other spinal column problems, improve and maintain good postural alignment, enhance proper and graceful body movement, improve personal appearance and self-image, and facilitate the development and maintenance of motor skills throughout life. Flexibility exercises have also been used successfully in the treatment of patients suffering from dysmenorrhea and general neuromuscular tension. Furthermore, stretching exercises in conjunction with calisthenics are helpful in warm-up routines to prepare the human body for more vigorous aerobic or strength-training exercises, as well as subsequent cool-down routines to help the organism return to the normal resting state.

Generally, during water aerobics, flexibility exercises are conducted after the toning exercises. Flexibility exercises are most effective when the person is properly warmed up. If the water temperature at your pool is cool, the flexibility phase should be done after the aerobic workout and prior to the toning exercises. Stretches should be held anywhere from 30 to 60 seconds — preferably 60 seconds — if the water temperature allows.

The Importance of Fun

Different things motivate different people to join and remain in a fitness program. Regardless of what the initial reason was for initiating the exercise program, you now need to plan for ways to make your class fun. The psychology behind it is simple. If you enjoy an activity, you will continue to do it. If you don't, you will quit. Some of the following suggestions may help:

1. Have a friend take the class with you. The social interaction will make exercise more fulfilling. Besides, it's harder to skip if someone else is waiting for you.

2. Socialize with others in class. Talk to your neighbor. Bring jokes to class.

3. Don't become a chronic exerciser. Learn to listen to your body. Overexercising can lead to chronic fatigue and injuries. Exercise should be enjoyable, and in the process you will need to "stop and smell the roses."

4. Exercise in different places and facilities (if feasible). This practice will add variety to your workouts.

5. Conduct periodic assessments. Improving to a higher fitness category is fun and a reward by itself.

6. Set realistic goals and share them with others. When you reach a particular goal, reward yourself with a new suit, other clothing, or buy something that you have wanted for a long time.

7. Develop your own methods (and share them with others) to make water aerobics an activity that you will want to continue for a lifetime.

WATER AEROBIC EXERCISES

The list and illustrations of exercises provided at the end of this chapter are for use in water aerobics. To make your selection easier, a list of all exercises and the phase of the workout where they can be used is provided in Table 3.1. Some of the warm-up and aerobic exercises can be used in either phase, depending on the intensity at which they are executed. Pre-stretch exercises (warm-up phase) and flexibility exercises are interchangeable as well, except that warm-up exercises are held for less than 30 seconds while flexibility exercises are held 30 to 60 seconds. You are encouraged to pre-stretch those areas that will be the most challenged during the aerobic phase of the workout.

To assist in the selection of exercises for your class, the aerobic phase exercises are subdivided into three different levels. Aerobic Level I exercises are recommended for beginners, Level II are for those who are reasonably fit, and Level III are for those who are highly fit.

Keep in mind that the intensity level during exercise can be modified by changing the tempo, the length of the lever, or the hand position (surface area). The intensity level that you select will be determined by your exercise heart rate. If you are below the target heart rate range, increase your intensity by lengthening the lever (arms) or increasing the surface area (changing your hand from a fist to a slightly cupped position). If you are above the target heart rate range, reduce the intensity by shortening the lever or changing the hand position. For all the exercises, unless specified otherwise, fold your hands in a paddle or slightly cupped position as shown in Figure 3.1.

SAMPLE CLASS SEQUENCE

The following is a sample class sequence for a 50-minute water aerobic class.

Phase	Exercise	Repetitions/ Counts Held	
Warm-up			
Isolation	Head Turn	2	
	Head Down	2	
	Shoulder Depressions/ Elevations	8	
	Alternating Shoulder Circles	8	
	Arm Circles Forward	8	
	Arm Circles Back	8	
	Torso Rotation	2	
	Knee Lifts	8	
	Rear Leg Lifts	8	
	Toe Jogs	8	
Actual Warm-up	The Russian	16	
	Biceps Curls	16	
	Press Downs	16	
	Pendulum Arms	16	
	Irish Jig	16	
	Pushdown Jump	16	
	Cross Country Skier	16	
Pre-stretch	Standing Calf	30	seconds
	Standing Hamstring	30	seconds
	Quad Stretch	30	seconds
	Back Lift	30	seconds
	Arm Across	30	seconds
Aerobic			
Gradual HR increase	Leap Right	8	
	Leap Left	8	
	Biceps Curl	16	
	Skater	16	
	Irish	16	
	Repeat all five above		
	Pushdown Jump	16	
	Skater	16	
	Straight Jump	16	
	Parallel Arms	16	
	Repeat all four above		
Actual Aerobic Phase	Froggies	16	
	Cross Country Skier	16	
	Straight Jump	16	
	Skater	16	
	Repeat all four above		

(continued on page 56)

SAMPLE CLASS SEQUENCE *(continued)*

Phase	Exercise	Repetitions/ Counts Held
	Cheerleader	16
	Cross Country Skier	16
	Pushdown Stride	16
	Cross Country Skier	16
	Repeat all four above	
	Cannonball	16
	Parallel Arms	16
	Donkey Kick	16
	Kick up Front	16
	Repeat all four above	
	"Lat" Pulls	16
	Cross Country Skier	16
	Eggbeater	16
	Cross Country Skier	16
	Repeat all four above	
	Row the Boat	16
	Kick up Front	16
	Jump Rope	16
	Cross Country	16
	Repeat all four above	
	Donkey Kicks	16
	Parallel Arms	16
	Jump Rope	16
	Cross Country Skier	16
	Repeat all four above	
	Straight Jump	16
	Skater	16
	Pushdown Jump	16
	Biceps Curl	16
	Repeat all four above	
Cool-down	Irish Jig	16
	Skater	16
	Pendulum Arms	16
	Heel Touches	16
	Repeat the above four but slowing down	
Toning	Hugs	3 sets of 15
	Golfer	3 sets of 15
	Figure 8	3 sets of 15
	Triceps Kickback	3 sets of 15
	Rotator Cuff	3 sets of 15
	Wash Windows	3 sets of 15
	Wrist Circles	3 sets of 15
Flexibility	Triceps	30–60 seconds
	Back Lift	30–60 seconds
	Indian	30–60 seconds
	Hamstring Wall Stretch	60 seconds
	Wall Calf Stretch	30–60 seconds

TABLE 3.1.

List of water aerobic exercises contained in this chapter
and workout phase in which they may be used.

	EXERCISE	PHASE
1.	Head Turn	Warm-up
2.	Head Down	Warm-up
3.	Shoulder Girdle Elevations	Warm-up
	and Depressions	Warm-up
4.	Alternating Shoulder Circles	Warm-up
5.	Arm Circles Forward	
	and Back	Warm-up
6.	Torso Rotation	Warm-up
7.	Knee Lifts	Warm-up
8.	Rear Leg Lifts	Warm-up
9.	Leg Lifts	Warm-up
10.	Toe Jogs	Warm-up
11.	Heel Touches	Warm-up
12.	Can Can	Warm-up
13.	The Russian	Warm-up
14.	Jumping Jacks	Warm-up
15.	Leaps	Warm-up, Aerobic I
16.	Bicep Curls	Warm-up, Aerobic I
17.	Press Downs	Warm-up, Aerobic I
18.	Jogging Hugs	Warm-up, Aerobic I
19.	Downward Hugs	Warm-up, Aerobic I
20.	Pendulum Arms	Warm-up, Aerobic I
21.	Climb the Wall	Warm-up, Aerobic I
22.	Elbow to Knee	Warm-up, Aerobic I
23.	Irish Jig	Warm-up, Aerobic I
24.	Skater	Warm-up, Aerobic I, II
25.	Eggbeater	Warm-up, Aerobic I, II, III
26.	Parallel Arms	Warm-up, Aerobic I, II, III
27.	Cross Country Skier	Warm-up, Aerobic I, II, III
28.	Pushdown Jump	Warm-up, Aerobic I, II
29.	Pushdown Stride	Warm-up, Aerobic I, II
30.	Straight Jump	Warm-up, Aerobic I, II,
31.	Froggies	Aerobic I, II
32.	Cheerleader	Aerobic I, II, III
33.	Row the Boat	Aerobic I, II, III
34.	"Lat" Pull	Aerobic I, II, III
35.	Weight Lift	Aerobic I, II, III
36.	Cannonball	Aerobic I, II, III
37.	Airborne Jumping Jacks	Aerobic I, II, III
38.	Kick up Front	Aerobic I, II, III

(continued on page 58)

TABLE 3.1. (continued)

EXERCISE	PHASE
39. Donkey Kick	Aerobic I, II, III
40. Jump Rope	Aerobic I, II, III
41. Rockers	Aerobic II, III
42. Deep Water Jog	Warm-up, Aerobic I, II, III
43. Deep Water Cross Country	Warm-up, Aerobic I, II, III
44. Neck Presses	Toning
45. Hugs	Toning
46. Golfer	Toning
47. Figure 8	Toning
48. Pendulums	Toning
49. Tricep Kickback	Toning
50. Push-ups	Toning
51. Squeezes	Toning
52. Wash Windows	Toning
53. Hand Squeezes	Toning
54. Wrist Circles	Toning
55. Rotator Cuff	Toning
56. Wall Curls	Toning
57. Side Leg Lift	Toning
58. Leg Pendulum	Toning
59. Leg Front and Backs	Toning
60. Flutter Kicks	Toning
61. Wall Scissors	Toning
62. Toe Taps	Toning
63. Ankle Circles	Toning
64. Bicycles	Toning
65. Milk Jug Leg Scissors	Toning
66. Milk Jug Strides	Toning
67. Milk Jug Flutters	Toning
68. Milk Jug Toe Taps	Toning
69. Milk Jug Ankle Circles	Toning
70. Milk Jug Quad and Hams	Toning
71. Milk Jug Bicycles	Toning
72. Standing Hamstring	Warm-up Pre-stretch, Flexibility
73. Standing Calf	Warm-up Pre-stretch, Flexibility
74. Quad Stretch	Warm-up Pre-stretch, Flexibility
75. Back Lift	Warm-up Pre-stretch, Flexibility
76. Arm Across	Warm-up Pre-stretch, Flexibility
77. Tricep	Warm-up Pre-stretch, Flexibility
78. Indian	Warm-up Pre-stretch, Flexibility

(continued on page 59)

TABLE 3.1. (continued)

EXERCISE	PHASE
79. Side Lift	Warm-up Pre-stretch, Flexibility
80. Shoulder Depressions	Flexibility
81. Wall Arm Stretch	Flexibility
82. Neck and Double Arm Stretch	Flexibility
83. Hamstring Wall Stretch	Flexibility
84. Wall Calf Stretch	Flexibility
85. Knee to Chest	Flexibility
86. Hip Flexor	Flexibility
87. Wall Straddle	Flexibility
88. Tailor	Flexibility

Exercise Tips

These water aerobic exercise tips have already been discussed in detail in this chapter. The following list is to be used as a reminder prior to exercise participation.

1. Always exercise at your own rate and under appropriate supervision.

2. To modify any of the exercises you may increase or decrease the following:
   a. height (range of motion) that the limbs are lifted.
   b. length of the lever arm(s).
   c. the tempo.
   d. the surface area.

3. During the performance of the exercises, unless otherwise specified, the hands should be held in a paddle or slightly cupped position (see Figure 3.1).

4. To prevent joint injuries you should keep the joints "soft." This implies that the joints should never be locked in place during any phase of the movements.

5. All movements during water exercises must be kept under control and the twisting actions should be limited to avoid potential injuries.

6. Be sure to always listen to your body. If a particular exercise causes you undue discomfort or pain, do not perform the exercise and check with your instructor.

7. Exercises 45, 46, 47, 48, 49, 51, 52, 54, and 55 can be performed with hand paddles. For an explanation on how to use hand paddles, refer to page 49.

8. Exercises 57, 58, and 59 can be performed with pull buoys. For an explanation on how to use pull buoys, refer to page 50.

9. Exercises 65 through 71 are for use with milk jugs. See page 51 for a description on how to use milk jugs.

10. Remember to HAVE FUN and make the most out of your water aerobics exercise program.

exercise 1

Head Turn

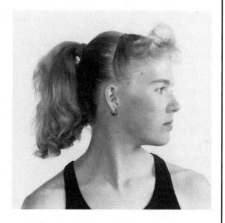

PHASE:
Warm-up, isolation

DESCRIPTION:
Begin with the head at the neutral position. Turn the head to look over the left shoulder and hold for two counts. Return to the center for two counts, turn toward the right shoulder and hold for two counts.

PRECAUTION: Keep the movement slow and pause at center or neutral position.

exercise 2

Head Down

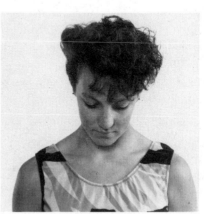

PHASE:
Warm-up, isolation

DESCRIPTION:
Begin with the head at the neutral position. Lower the head toward the chest and hold for two counts. Return to neutral and hold for two counts.

PRECAUTION:
Keep the motion slow, pausing at the neutral position. Do not take the head to the rear or hyperextended position because vertigo or neck injury could result.

exercise 3

Shoulder Girdle Elevations and Depressions

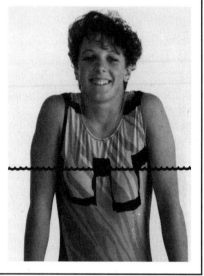

PHASE:
Warm-up, isolation

DESCRIPTION:
Elevate the shoulders toward the ears and return, pausing at the neutral position. Depress the shoulders and return to the neutral position.

exercise 4

Alternating Shoulder Circles

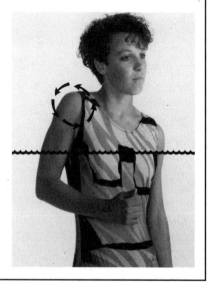

PHASE:
Warm-up, isolation

DESCRIPTION:
Circle the right shoulder toward the back. When it is at the back and in the down position, circle the left shoulder back. Continue in an alternating fashion, increasing the circle size, and gradually adding the upper arm (keep the forearm flexed).

PRECAUTIONS:
Begin with a small range of motion and gradually increase the size of the circle.

exercise 5

Arm Circles Forward and Back

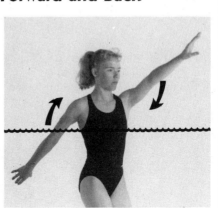

PHASE:
Warm–up, isolation

DESCRIPTION:
Begin with the right arm. Lift the arm upward to the rear while keeping the elbow joint soft. Circle it slowly to the front. When the right arm reaches the forward position, begin lifting the left arm upward and to the rear. Continue in an alternating fashion increasing the circle size.

PRECAUTION: Keep the action slow and begin with a small range of motion. To prevent injuries, forward circles should be done before rear circles.

exercise 6

Torso Rotation

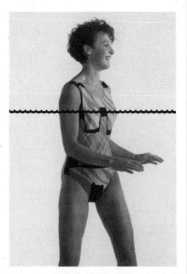

PHASE:
Warm–up, isolation

DESCRIPTION:
Stand with knees slightly flexed. Begin by twisting the upper part of your torso to the left and hold for two counts. Return to the forward position for two counts, and repeat to the right.

PRECAUTION:
Hips and knees should not move from the forward facing position. The twist should come from the torso only. The pace should be slow.

exercise 7

Knee Lifts

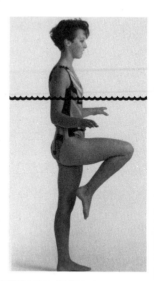

PHASE:
Warm-up, isolation

DESCRIPTION:
Stand with hands at your sides. Lift the right knee to the front, flexing the lower leg. Pause, then set it down. Repeat with the left knee.

PRECAUTION/MODIFICATION:
Begin with a small range of motion. To prevent back strain, the knees should not be lifted higher than the waist. To modify the exercise, reduce the height that the knee is lifted.

VARIATION:
Repeat the exercise lifting the knees to the side.

exercise 8

Rear Leg Lifts

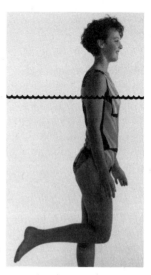

PHASE:
Warm-up, isolation

DESCRIPTION:
From the standing position pick up the right leg and bend it at the knee, lifting the foot toward the back. Return to the starting position. Repeat with the left leg.

PRECAUTION/MODIFICATION:
Begin with a small range of motion. For those who may have knee problems, reduce the foot lift to 90 degrees.

exercise 9

Leg Lifts

PHASE:
Warm-up, isolation

DESCRIPTION:
Standing with hands out to the side, lift the right leg up to the front. The knee should be kept slightly flexed. Return to the starting position and repeat with the left leg.

PRECAUTION/MODIFICATION:
Begin with a small range of motion and do not lift the leg above waist level. To modify the exercise, reduce the height that the leg is lifted.

VARIATION:
Lift the legs diagonally to the side.

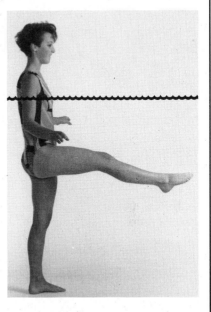

exercise 10

Toe Jogs

PHASE:
Warm-up, isolation

DESCRIPTION:
Begin with both feet on the ground. Raise the heel of the right foot, keeping the toe in contact with the ground. As you lower the right heel back to the ground raise the left heel up. Continue alternating the action.

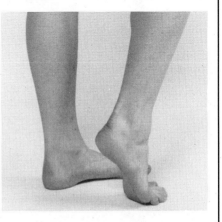

PRECAUTION: Slowly roll the foot down to the ground.

exercise 11

Heel Touches

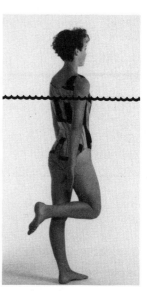

PHASE:
Warm-up

DESCRIPTION:
Jog, lifting your heels toward your buttock. Alternate touching the right heel to the right hand and the left heel to the left hand.

MODIFICATION:
Reduce the height that the foot is lifted.

VARIATION:
Repeat the same leg action only diagonally back and to the side.

exercise 12

Can Can

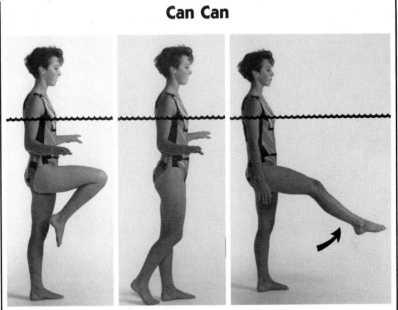

PHASE: Warm-up

DESCRIPTION: Raise the right knee up to the front flexing the lower leg. Touch the right foot back down to the ground. Lift the same leg back up and kick the foot out to the front. Return the leg back to the starting position. Repeat with the left leg.

PRECAUTION/MODIFICATION: To protect the knee, keep the joint soft. To modify the exercise, limit the height that the leg is lifted.

VARIATION: Repeat the same action, using a forward diagonal motion.

exercise **13**
The Russian

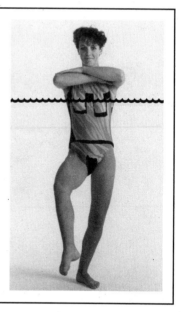

PHASE:
Warm-up

DESCRIPTION:
With the arms crossed at chest level, jog, lifting your legs 45 degrees toward the front. Turn the toes slightly out.

PRECAUTION/MODIFICATION:
Keep the knee joint soft. To modify the exercise, reduce the height that the leg is lifted.

exercise **14**
Jumping Jack

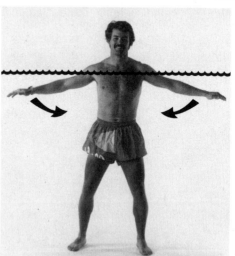

PHASE:
Warm-up

DESCRIPTION:
Stand with feet together and arms down at sides. Jump to a straddled-leg position and at the same time lift your arms up to the side horizontally. Jump back to the starting position pressing the arms down to the sides.

PRECAUTION/ MODIFICATION: To prevent stress on the knee joint, limit the width of the straddle position.

exercise 15

Leaps

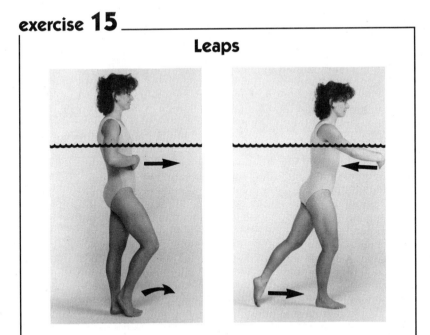

PHASE: Warm-up, aerobic I

DESCRIPTION: Begin with elbows flexed and the hands touching your abdomen. Leap to the right with the right leg, while extending the arms with the wrists at 90 degrees. When you land on the right foot, bring the left leg toward it. At the same time flex the arms, bringing the hands back to the starting position. Reverse the leg action when moving to the left.

PRECAUTION: To prevent hyperextension of the low back, keep abdominal muscles tight.

exercise 16 _____
Bicep Curls

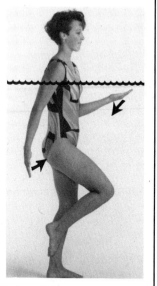

PHASE:
Warm-up, aerobic I

DESCRIPTION:
Begin with arms at the sides. Jog in place
and flex the left arm at the elbow. Bring
the hand up toward the surface. Flex the
right arm toward the surface as you
extend the left arm back to the starting
position. Repeat in an alternating
fashion. The right leg should be flexed
when the left arm is bent and vice versa.

PRECAUTION:
Keep the tempo slow enough so that the
entire action can be completed. Hands
should be kept in the water at all times.
Keep the elbow joints soft when in extended position.

exercise 17 _____
Press Downs

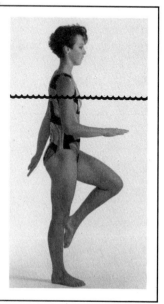

PHASE:
Warm-up, aerobic I

DESCRIPTION:
Begin with the arms at the sides. Flex the
right arm at the elbow toward the front.
Keep the palm down. Flex the left arm
in the same manner as you extend the
right back to the starting position. Add a
jog to these actions.

PRECAUTION:
Keep the tempo slow. Hands should be
kept in the water at all times. Keep the
elbow joints soft.

exercise 18

Jogging Hugs

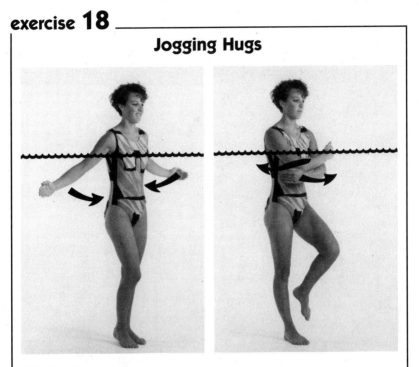

PHASE: Warm-up, aerobic I

DESCRIPTION: Begin with both arms held out at your side, below the surface of the water. Palms should face forward. As you jog, hug the water, pressing both arms forward, wrapping the arms around the body. Return to the starting position.

PRECAUTION: To create greater resistance, keep the arms below the surface of the water. Elbow joints should be kept soft.

exercise 19

Downward Hugs

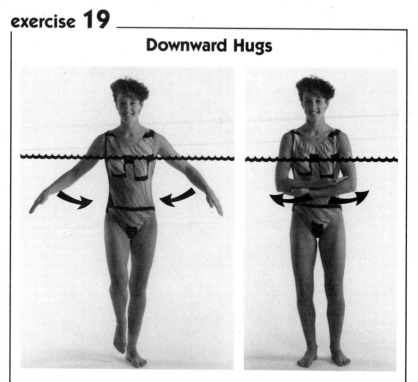

PHASE: Warm-up, aerobic I

DESCRIPTION: Begin with your arms held out to the side, under the water, palms facing the bottom. Jog and hug the water pressing down. When your hands are in front of your thighs flex both forearms bringing your palms up. Reverse the procedure back to the starting position.

PRECAUTION: Keep your elbow joints soft when you return to the starting position.

exercise 20
Pendulum Arms

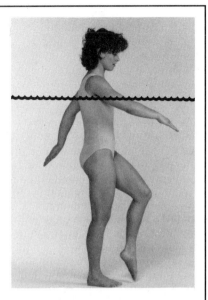

PHASE:
Warm-up, aerobic I

DESCRIPTION:
Begin with your arms at the sides with palms facing back. As you jog, lift the right arm 45 degrees to the front. At the same time press the left arm 45 degrees to the back. Continue to alternate the action. The left leg should be lifted when the right arm is forward and vice versa.

PRECAUTION:
Elbow joints should be kept soft and hands should remain in the water.

exercise 21
Climb the Wall

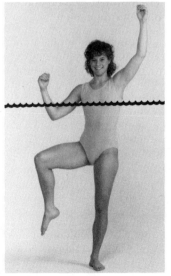

PHASE:
Warm-up, aerobic I

DESCRIPTION:
Begin in a standing position with the arms flexed and hands touching the shoulders. Jump to the left foot, lifting the right knee diagonally to the side. At the same time lower the right elbow toward the knee as the left arms extends upward. Reverse the action and repeat the exercise.

PRECAUTION/MODIFICATION:
To protect the back, limit the height of the knee lift. The exercise can be modified by reducing the arm extension or eliminating the action entirely.

exercise 22

Elbow to Knee

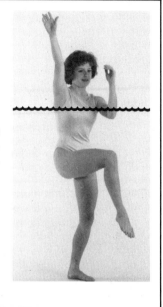

PHASE:
Warm-up, aerobic I

DESCRIPTION:
From a standing position, flex the arms and touch the hands to the shoulders. With the weight on the left foot, lift the right knee and simultaneously bring the left elbow down toward the right knee, while extending the right arm upward. Reverse the action, jumping onto the right foot.

PRECAUTION/MODIFICATION:
To protect the low back, limit the height of the knee lifts. To modify the arm action, keep them in the water or reduce the height of the arm extension.

exercise 23

Irish Jig

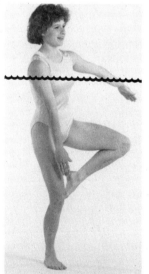

PHASE:
Warm-up, aerobic I

DESCRIPTION:
Hold the arms out horizontally to the left side with the palms facing each other. Hop on the right foot and bend the left knee, bringing the left foot up to the mid-line of the body. At the same time, bring the right arm down to the front and touch the left heel in front of the body. Repeat the action using the right foot and the left arm.

PRECAUTION:
Keep the knee lifts below the waist to protect the back.

VARIATION: Use the same actions, but lift the heel backward and touch the heel behind you.

exercise 24

Skater

PHASE:
Warm-up, aerobic I and II

DESCRIPTION:
Jog side to side, lifting your feet up to the rear. With the weight on your left foot, extend the left arm horizontally out to the side with the palm down. At the same time flex the right elbow down. Alternate the arm actions when the right foot is in contact with the bottom of the pool.

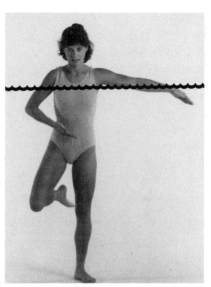

PRECAUTION:
For those with knee problems, reduce the height that the leg is lifted.

exercise 25

Eggbeater

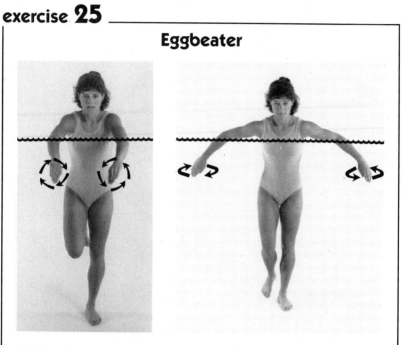

PHASE: Warm-up, aerobic I, II, and III

DESCRIPTION: Jog in place and circle the arms to the center, out, and around. The same action can be done but circling in the opposite direction.

PRECAUTION: Keep the arm circles small and the arms under water.

exercise **26**

Parallel Arms

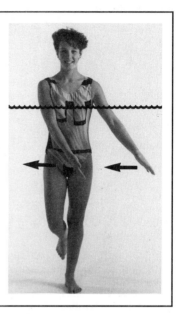

PHASE:
Warm-up, aerobic I, II, and III

DESCRIPTION:
Jog in place and begin with the arms down in front and to the left with palms facing each other. Press the arms to the opposite side.

PRECAUTION:
For back protection, keep the abdomen muscles tight and do not allow the torso to twist.

exercise **27**

Cross Country Skier

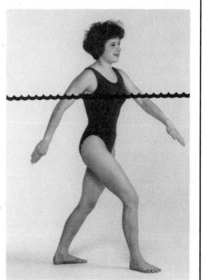

PHASE:
Warm-up, aerobic I, II, and III

DESCRIPTION:
Begin in a stride position with the right leg forward. The left arm is also forward at a 45-degree angle, while the right arm is back to the rear at 45 degrees. Both palms face backward. Jump and switch the arm and leg positions.

PRECAUTION:
Keep arms straight and the elbow joints soft.

VARIATION: Use the same leg action with the parallel arms described in exercise #26.

exercise 28

Pushdown Jump

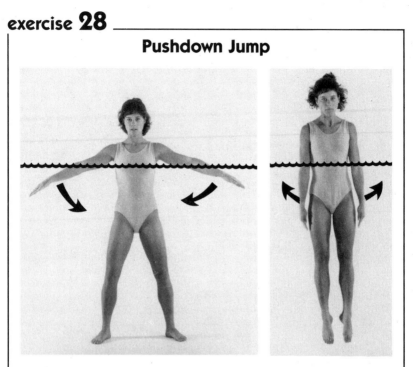

PHASE: Warm-up, aerobic I and II

DESCRIPTION: Begin with arms held horizontally out to the side with the palms down. Jump up and at the same time press your arms down all the way to the thighs. Lift the arms back to horizontal as you return to standing position. Do not raise the arms out of the water.

PRECAUTION: Reduce the height of the jump to modify this exercise.

exercise **29**
Pushdown Stride

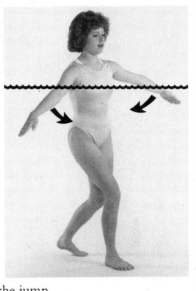

PHASE:
Warm-up, aerobic I and II

DESCRIPTION:
Begin in a stride position with the right foot forward, the arms held out horizontally to the side, and the palms down. Jump and switch the legs while pressing the arms down to the sides. Lift the arms back to horizontal as you land.

PRECAUTION/MODIFICATION:
Keep the stride position narrow to maintain balance. To modify the exercise reduce the height of the jump.

exercise **30**
Straight Jump

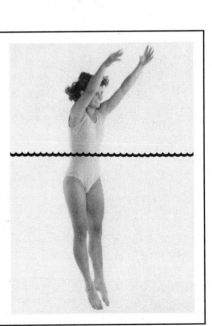

PHASE:
Warm-up, aerobic I and II

DESCRIPTION:
With arms bent and held in front of your body, jump straight up extending your arms up in front of you. Return the arms to the starting position as you land.

MODIFICATION:
You can modify the exercise by reducing the height that the arms are raised or you may also leave them in the water.

exercise 31
Froggies

PHASE:
Aerobic I and II

DESCRIPTION:
Start with the elbows bent and the hands facing at chest level. Jump up bringing both knees diagonally forward to the sides. At the same time, press the hands down the mid-line of the body. Return to the starting position before landing.

PRECAUTION/MODIFICATION:
Keep the knees below waist level to protect the back. Modify the exercise by varying the height that the knees are lifted.

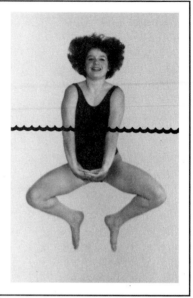

exercise 32
Cheerleader Jump

PHASE:
Aerobic I, II, and III

DESCRIPTION:
Begin in a standing position, hands touching the shoulders. Jump up and move the feet to a straddle position and at the same time extend the forearms up and diagonally forward. Bring the feet together and hands back to the shoulders before landing.

PRECAUTION/MODIFICATION:
Keep the arm action controlled. To modify the exercise: (a) reduce the arm range of motion or keep the arms in the water at all times and (b) narrow the width of the straddle position.

exercise 33
Row the Boat

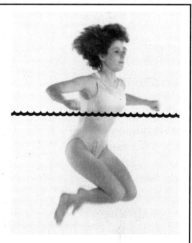

PHASE:
Aerobic I, II, and III

DESCRIPTION:
Start with the arms held horizontally out in front of the body. Jump and bring both knees up to the front, at the same time pulling the arms back toward the chest (imitating a rowing action). Return to the starting position prior before landing.

PRECAUTION/MODIFICATION:
The knees should be kept below the waist to protect the back. Modify the exercise by eliminating or lowering the arm action, and/or reducing the height that the knees are raised.

exercise 34
"Lat" Pull

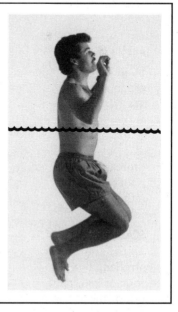

PHASE:
Aerobic I, II, and III

DESCRIPTION:
Begin with the arms extended over the head and slightly in front of the body. Jump and bring both knees up to the front while pulling the arms down toward eye level. Return to the starting position before you land.

PRECAUTION/MODIFICATION:
Keep the hands in front of the body and knees below the waist. Modify the "lat" pull by eliminating or lowering the arm action, and/or reducing the height that the knees are raised.

exercise 35

Weight Lift

PHASE:
Aerobic I, II, and III

DESCRIPTION:
Begin with the hands at the
sides. Jump and bring both
knees to the front while lifting
the arms up to waist level at the
sides. Return to the starting
position for landing.

PRECAUTION/MODIFICATION:
Keep the knees below the waist
for back protection. To modify
the exercise reduce the amount
of knee lift.

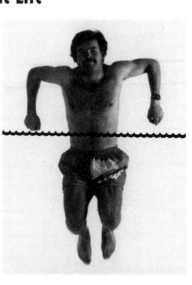

exercise 36

Cannonball

PHASE:
Aerobic I, II, and III

DESCRIPTION:
Begin with hands touching the
shoulders. As you jump, bring
both knees up to the front, while
reaching down and touching the
hands to the knees. Return to the
starting position for landing.

PRECAUTION/MODIFICATION:
To protect the lower back, knees
should remain below waist level.
To modify the exercise, reduce the
knee lift and eliminate or reduce
the arm action.

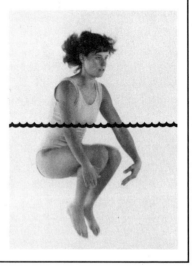

exercise 37
Airborne Jumping Jacks

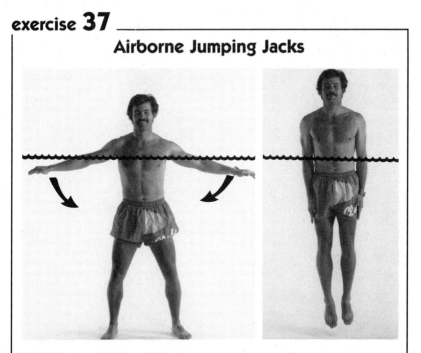

PHASE: Aerobic II and III

DESCRIPTION: Begin with the hands held horizontally out to the sides and the legs in a straddle position. Jump up bringing the legs together and pressing the arms to the sides. Return to the starting position for landing.

PRECAUTION/MODIFICATION: Keep the straddle position narrow. Modify the exercise by reducing the height of the jump.

exercise **38**
Kick-Up Front

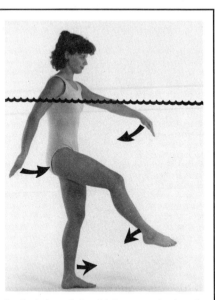

PHASE:
Aerobic I, II, and III

DESCRIPTION:
Hop on the left foot while kicking the right foot forward 45 degrees. At the same time press the left hand forward 45 degrees and the right hand back 45 degrees. The palms of the hand should face backward. Hop to the right foot and at the same time reverse the arm and leg position.

PRECAUTION/MODIFICATION:
For back protection, keep the knees slightly flexed and limit the height of the kick to waist level. Modify the exercise by reducing the height of the kick.

exercise **39**
Donkey Kick

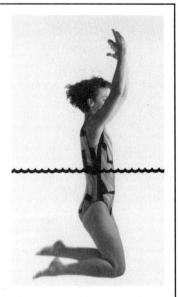

PHASE:
Aerobic I, II, and III

DESCRIPTION:
Begin with hands on the shoulders. Jump and lift the feet toward the back while extending the arms up to the front. Return to the starting position for landing.

PRECAUTION/MODIFICATION:
Keep the abdominal muscles tight and lift the feet no more than 90 degrees. To modify the exercise, eliminate or reduce the arm action.

exercise 40
Jump Rope

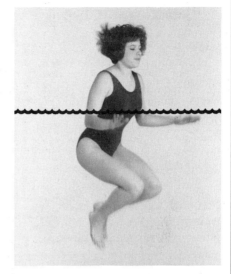

PHASE:
Aerobic I, II, and III

DESCRIPTION:
Jump and bring the knees to the front while circling the forearms forward, down and around, similar to twirling a rope. This exercise can also be done by circling the arms to the rear.

PRECAUTION:
Keep the knees below the waist to protect the back.

exercise 41
Rockers

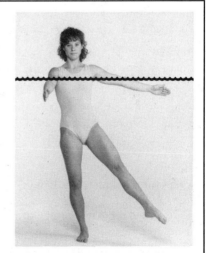

PHASE:
Aerobic II and III

DESCRIPTION:
Begin with the arms held below the surface of the water. Hold the left arm out horizontally to the side and the right arm horizontally to the front. The palms should face each other. Hop to the right foot, kicking the left leg diagonally to the side. At the same time press the arms diagonally to the right. Switch the arm and leg action as you hop to the left foot.

PRECAUTION: To protect the back, the inside arm should not cross the midline of the body and the legs should not be lifted above 45 degrees.

exercise 42
Deep Water Jog

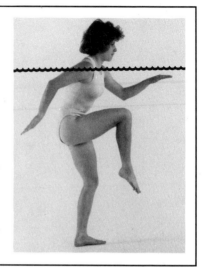

PHASE:
Warm-up, aerobic I, II and III

DESCRIPTION:
Bend the torso forward and combine a jogging action with an alternating arm-pumping action. Palms should face down.

PRECAUTION:
To protect the knees, do not fully extend the knee joint at any time.

exercise 43
Deep Water Cross Country

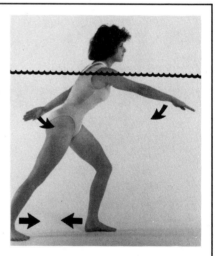

PHASE:
Warm-up, aerobic I, II, and III

DESCRIPTION:
Bend the torso forward and use an alternating pendulum action with the arms, combined with an alternating forward and backward leg stride. The palms of the hand face backward. The opposite arm and leg are forward at the same time.

PRECAUTION: Keep the knee joint soft when the leg is extended.

★ The above two exercises should be done only with lifeguard supervision and require intermediate swimming skills. A specialized vest ("wet-vest") for extra support can also be purchased for use with these exercises.

exercise 44
Neck Presses

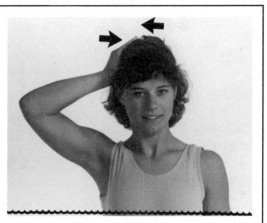

PHASE:
Toning

DESCRIPTION:
Stand and place the
right hand against
the right side of the
head. While keeping
the head in the neutral
position, tense the
neck muscles and
press against the
resisting hand. Hold the tension for 10 counts. Repeat using the left
hand for the left side. Use both hands for front and back resistance.

PRECAUTION: Keep the head in the neutral position at all times.

exercise 45
Hugs

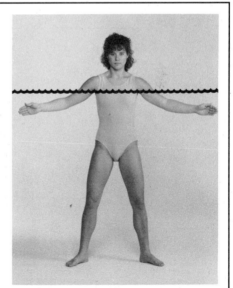

PHASE:
Toning

DESCRIPTION:
Stand in chest deep water,
feet apart and knees slightly
bent. Begin with the arms
held out to the side and the
palms facing forward. Hug
the water, wrapping the
arms around the body.
Reverse the action, unwrap-
ping the arms and ending in
the starting position.

VARIATION:
Use the same procedure,
only press downward.

PRECAUTION: Keep the elbows slightly flexed when returning to
the starting position.

exercise **46**
Golfer

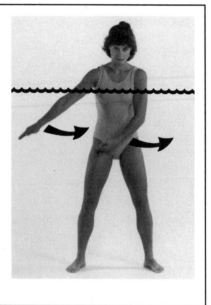

PHASE:
Toning

DESCRIPTION:
Stand in chest deep water with the feet apart and knees slightly bent. Keep the shoulders and hips square. Lift both arms diagonally to the right side with the palms facing each other. Press the arms down and over to the left side and then return to the starting position.

PRECAUTION:
For back protection keep the hips and shoulders square.

exercise **47**
Figure 8

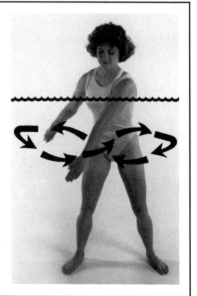

PHASE:
Toning

DESCRIPTION:
Stand in chest deep water with the feet apart and knees slightly bent. Lift both arms diagonally to the right side, keeping them in the water, and palms facing each other. Keep the hips and shoulders square as you press the arms through the water in a figure eight pattern.

PRECAUTION:
Tighten the abdominal muscles to prevent twisting of the back.

exercise 48
Pendulums

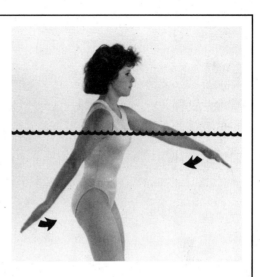

PHASE:
Toning

DESCRIPTION:
Stand in chest deep water with the legs slightly flexed. Press the left arm forward 45 degrees and the right arm backward 45 degrees. The palms should face backward. Repeat alternating the arm motion.

PRECAUTION: Keep the elbow joints soft.

exercise 49
Tricep Kickbacks

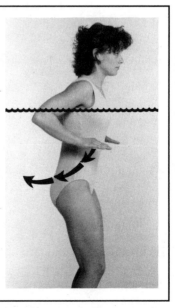

PHASE:
Toning

DESCRIPTION:
Stand in chest deep water with the legs slightly flexed. Lean forward with the torso. Begin with the palms facing down and the forearms flexed 90 degrees. Press down and back with the forearm. Return to the starting position.

PRECAUTION:
Keep the elbow joints soft when in the extended position.

exercise 50
Push-Ups

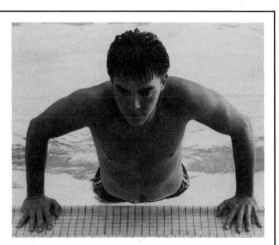

PHASE:
Toning

DESCRIPTION:
Stand in waist deep water and place the hands on the side of the pool (shoulder width apart). Slowly lift your body out of the water until your arms are fully extended. Slowly lower yourself back to the starting position.

PRECAUTION/MODIFICATION: During the exercise, do not lean against the side of the pool. A small jump can be added for those who have difficulty pressing up.

exercise 51
Squeezes

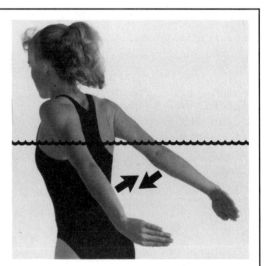

PHASE:
Toning

DESCRIPTION:
Stand in chest deep water with the legs slightly flexed and the torso leaning forward. Extend the arms diagonally down to the back with palms facing. Squeeze the shoulder blades together moving the hands toward each other. Return to the starting position.

PRECAUTION: Keep the arm movement small. Concentrate on using the upper back muscles as opposed to the arms.

exercise 52 _____

Window Wash

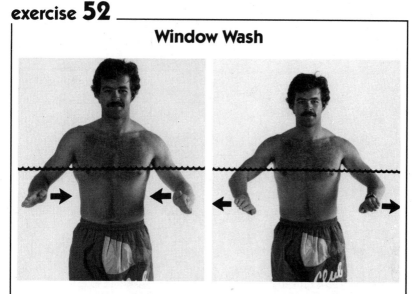

PHASE: Toning

DESCRIPTION: Stand in chest deep water with your legs slightly flexed. Hold the arms in front of you with the elbows bent and the palms down. Draw both hands in to the center with the palms angled up toward each other (thumbs up). Now press the hands back out, rotating the thumbs down, pushing the palms away from each other. The entire action should be performed rapidly.

exercise **53**

Hand Squeezes

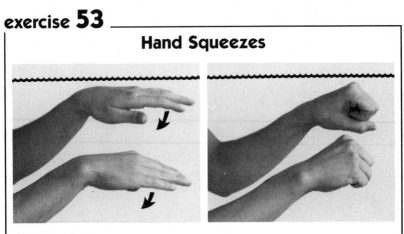

PHASE: Toning

DESCRIPTION: Stand in chest deep water with the arms held in front of you with the palms down. Now fully close the hands as though you were grabbing the water, followed by complete extension and spreading of the fingers. Repeat this action rapidly.

exercise **54**

Wrist Circles

PHASE:
Toning

DESCRIPTION:
In chest deep water, flex the elbows in front of you, keeping the hands under the water. Perform wrists circles clockwise and repeat the action counterclockwise.

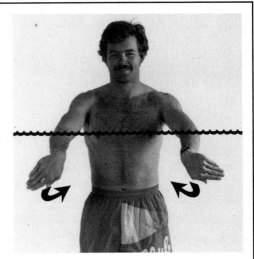

exercise 55

Rotator Cuff

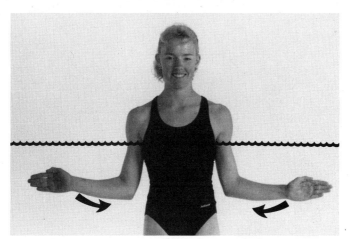

PHASE:
Toning

DESCRIPTION:
Stand in chest deep water with the legs slightly flexed. Begin with the elbows near the sides of the body, the forearms held out horizontally, and palms facing forward. Press the hands forward, crossing all the way to the opposite side. Return to the starting position.

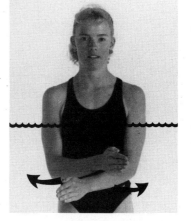

Be sure to keep the elbows near the sides of the body during the entire exercise.

PRECAUTION: Control the arm action at all times.

exercise 56

Wall Curls

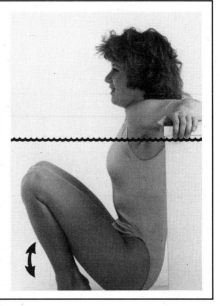

PHASE:
Toning

DESCRIPTION:
With the back to the pool wall, brace yourself by extending the arms along the edge. Begin with the knees bent at 90 degrees and the small of your back (lower back) pressed against the wall. Slowly curl the knees up until they reach the surface of the water. Lower the knees back down to the starting position.

exercise 57

Side Leg Lift

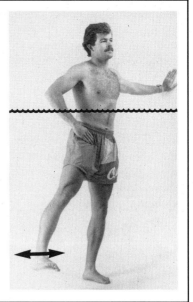

PHASE:
Toning

DESCRIPTION:
Support yourself with your left hand at the edge of the pool with the left side to the pool wall. Place your weight on the left foot and press the right leg out to the side to a 45 degree angle. Return to the starting position. Switch the position for left leg sets.

PRECAUTION:
Keep both knee joints soft and the toes pointed forward. Do not raise the leg higher than 45 degrees.

exercise 58 _____

Leg Pendulum

PHASE:
Toning

DESCRIPTION:
Support yourself with your left
hand while standing with the left
side to the pool wall. With the
weight on the left leg, both knees
slightly flexed, and the abdominal
muscles tight, press the right leg
forward and back to a 15 degree
angle in both directions. Switch
the position for left leg sets.

PRECAUTION/MODIFICATION:
Keep the knee joints soft and the
abdominal muscles tight. To
modify the exercise, reduce the
height that the leg is lifted.

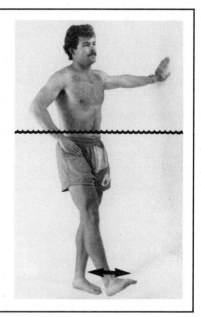

exercise 59 _____

Leg Front and Backs

PHASE:
Toning

DESCRIPTION:
Support yourself with your right
hand and your right side to the
wall. Begin with the weight on the
right foot and hold the left foot out
in front. While keeping the toes
pointed forward, press the left leg
out and around in an arc, ending
with the left foot behind the right.
Return to the starting position,
reversing the arc. Switch positions
for right leg sets.

PRECAUTION:
Keep both knee joints soft,
abdominal muscles tight, and toes
pointed forward. Keep the size of the arc small.

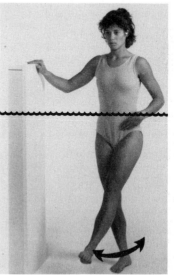

exercise 60

Flutter Kicks

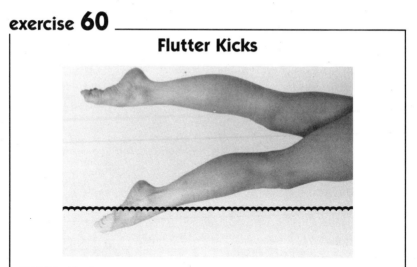

PHASE: Toning

DESCRIPTION: With the back against the wall and the arms along the pool edge, allow the legs to float up toward the surface. Keep the legs straight and the toes pointed, while kicking the legs up and down in an alternating fashion.

PRECAUTION: Keep the knee joints soft during the entire action.

exercise 61

Wall Scissors

PHASE:
Toning

DESCRIPTION:
Brace yourself with the back against the wall and the arms along the pool edge. Press the lower back

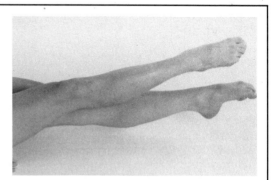

to the wall, lift the legs up to the front to a 45 degree angle in a straddle position. Press the legs toward the center, crossing the feet and then return to the starting position.

PRECAUTION: Keep the lower back pressed against the wall during the entire exercise. Knee joints should remain soft.

exercise 62
Toe Taps

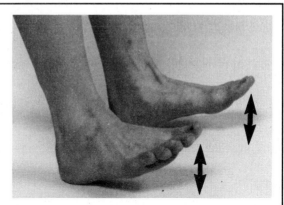

PHASE:
Toning

DESCRIPTION:
Stand, supporting
yourself with the
back to the wall.
While holding the
heels on the
bottom of the
pool, lift the toes
as high as possible. Tap the toes up and down.

VARIATION: Repeat the same action tapping the feet in an arc, out
and then in.

exercise 63
Ankle Circles

PHASE: Toning

DESCRIPTION: Support yourself with the left side to the wall and the
weight on the left foot. Lift the right leg off the bottom of the pool
and circle the ankle around clockwise. Repeat the action moving the
ankle counterclockwise. Switch the supporting position for the left
leg.

exercise 64
Bicycles

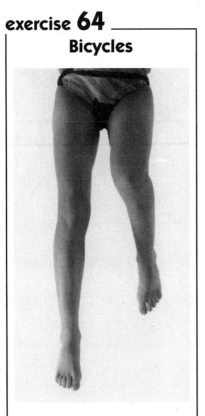

PHASE: Toning

DESCRIPTION: Begin with the back to the wall and the arms along the pool edge. The legs are held out horizontally. Turn the hips to the right and perform a pedaling action with your legs. Repeat the action with the hips turned to the left.

PRECAUTION: To protect the knees, keep the knee joints soft during the entire action.

exercise 65*
Milk Jug Leg Scissors

PHASE: Toning

DESCRIPTION: Begin with the legs suspended straight down. Straddle the legs diagonally out to a 45-degree angle. Return them back to the starting position, crossing one foot in front of the other.

PRECAUTION: Keep the knee joints soft at all times.

* For exercises 65-71 see explanation on milk jugs on page 51.

exercise 66
Milk Jug Strides

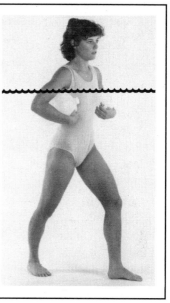

PHASE:
Toning

DESCRIPTION:
Begin with the legs hanging vertically.
Press the left leg forward and the right
leg backward to 45-degree angles
(large strides). Switch the position in
an alternating or walking fashion.

PRECAUTION:
Keep the knee joints soft.

exercise 67
Milk Jug Flutters

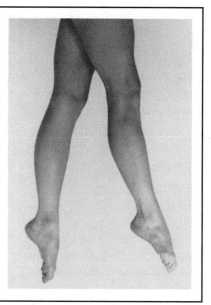

PHASE:
Toning

DESCRIPTION:
Begin with the legs hanging
vertically. Kick the legs in an
alternating forward and backward motion, but only use a
small range of motion.

PRECAUTION:
Keep the knee joints soft during
the entire exercise.

exercise 68

Milk Jug
Toe Taps

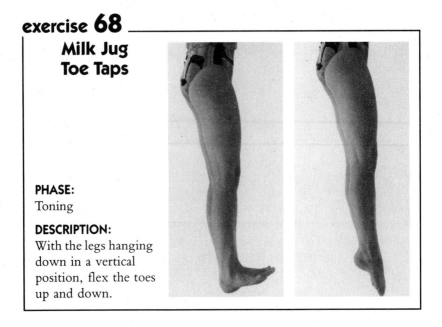

PHASE:
Toning

DESCRIPTION:
With the legs hanging
down in a vertical
position, flex the toes
up and down.

exercise 69

Milk Jug
Ankle Circles

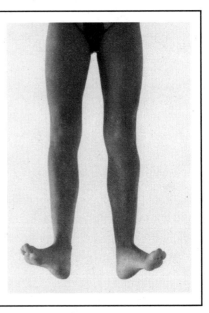

PHASE:
Toning

DESCRIPTION:
While hanging in a vertical
position, circle both ankles to
the outside. Repeat the action
circling the ankles to the inside.

exercise 70
Milk Jug Quad and Hams

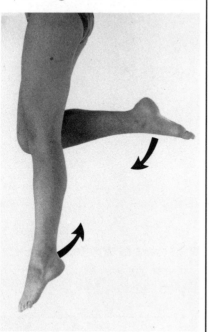

PHASE: Toning

DESCRIPTION: Begin by flexing the right leg back to a 90 degree angle and keep the left leg straight. Now flex the left knee 90 degrees and at the same time extend the right leg. Continue in alternating fashion.

PRECAUTION: Keep the knee joints soft when in the extended position.

exercise 71
Milk Jug Bicycles

PHASE: Toning

DESCRIPTION: Begin in a vertical hanging position and pedal as though you were riding a bicycle. This exercise can also be done in a side lying position.

exercise 72
Standing Hamstring

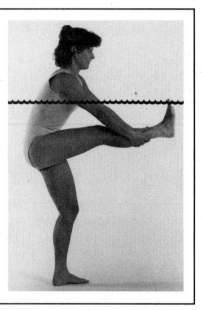

PHASE:
Warm-up prestretch, flexibility

DESCRIPTION:
Stand on one leg, lift the opposite leg and grasp it with both hands near the ankle. Gently extend the leg forward until you feel it stretch. Hold the stretch for 10 to 60 seconds. Repeat with opposite leg.

PRECAUTION:
Keep the knee joints soft. To reduce the tension, flex the knee joint.

exercise 73
Standing Calf Stretch

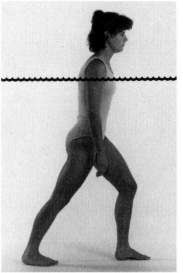

PHASE:
Warm-up prestretch, flexibility

DESCRIPTION:
Stand in a stride position with the back leg straight. Turn the rear foot slightly inward and press the heel toward the bottom of the pool. Hold for 10 to 60 seconds. Now, flex the knee of the back leg and once again press the heel down. Hold for 10 to 60 seconds. Repeat with the opposite leg.

PRECAUTION/MODIFICATION:
The stretch should be slightly uncomfortable, but not painful. To modify the exercise reduce the tension.

exercise 74

Quad Stretch

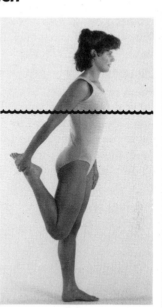

PHASE:
Warm-up prestretch, flexibility

DESCRIPTION:
Stand on the left leg and flex the right leg backward. Grasp the foot (where your shoelaces would be) with the right hand. Keep the abdominal muscles tight and the torso erect. Now gently extend the right thigh backward. Hold for 10 to 60 seconds. Repeat for the left leg.

PRECAUTION:
To prevent back injury, avoid leaning forward. To prevent knee injury, do not pull the foot toward the buttock, instead push the thigh backward.

exercise 75

Backlift

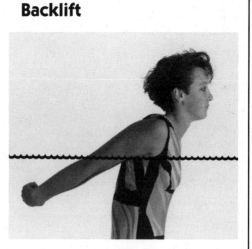

PHASE:
Warm-up prestretch, flexibility

DESCRIPTION:
Grasp the hands together behind the back. Keep the knees slightly flexed and bend the head and torso forward. Gently lift (press) the arms upward. Hold for 10 to 60 seconds.

exercise 76

Arm Across

PHASE:
Warm-up prestretch,
flexibility

DESCRIPTION:
Bring the right arm across
the front of the body at
shoulder height. Grasp above
the right elbow with the left
hand. Gently pull the arm
across the body. Hold for 10
to 60 seconds. Repeat with
the left arm.

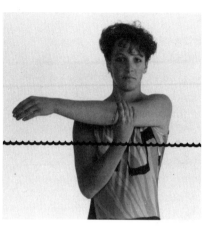

PRECAUTION:
Do not pull too hard to prevent injury to the shoulder joint.

exercise 77

Tricep

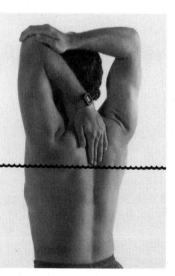

PHASE:
Warm-up prestretch, flexibility

DESCRIPTION:
Place the left hand behind the head.
Grasp the left arm above the elbow
with the right hand. Gently pull
the elbow backward. Hold for 10
to 60 seconds. Switch positions
and repeat for the right arm.

exercise 78

Indian

PHASE:
Warm-up prestretch, flexibility

DESCRIPTION:
Fold the arms in front of you at shoulder height. Press the elbows forward and hold for 10 to 60 seconds.

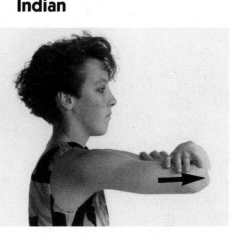

exercise 79

Side Lift

PHASE:
Warm-up prestretch, flexibility

DESCRIPTION:
Raise the left arm, lift up with the chest, and reach toward the right side. Hold the stretch for 10 to 60 seconds. Switch positions and repeat with the right arm up.

PRECAUTION:
To protect the back, lift the chest up as opposed to just bending the body to the side.

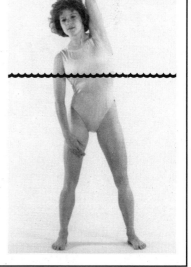

exercise 80

Shoulder Depressions

PHASE:
Flexibility

DESCRIPTION:
Stand in a relaxed position. Depress the right shoulder and at the same time press the head toward the left. Hold for 10 to 60 seconds. Repeat with the other shoulder.

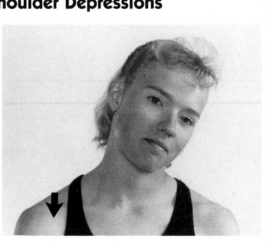

exercise 81

Wall Arm Stretch

PHASE:
Flexibility

DESCRIPTION:
Stand with the right side of the body to the pool wall. Hold on to the edge of the pool with the right hand and then slowly turn toward the left. Stop when you feel the stretch and hold this position from 10 to 60 seconds. Repeat the exercise with the opposite side.

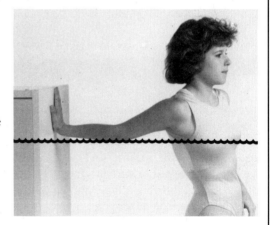

exercise 82 _____

Neck and Double Arm Stretch

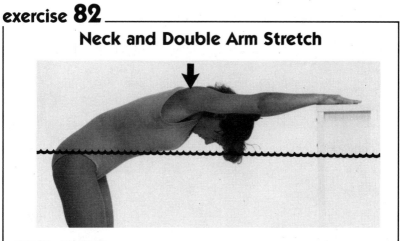

PHASE: Flexibility

DESCRIPTION: Bend at the waist and place both arms on the edge of the pool. Now lower the head between the arms until you begin to feel tension. Hold the stretch for 10 to 60 seconds. This stretch can also be done against a wall if the pool does not have a raised edge.

exercise 83 _____

Hamstring Wall Stretch

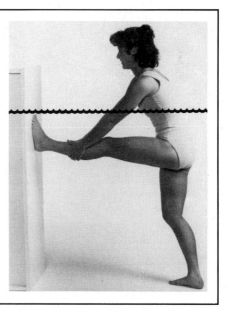

PHASE:
Flexibility

DESCRIPTION:
Place the left leg against a wall or edge of the pool. With the leg straight, slowly press the torso forward toward the leg. Hold for 10 to 60 seconds. Repeat for the right leg.

PRECAUTION:
Keep the knee joints of both legs soft.

exercise 84
Wall Calf Stretch

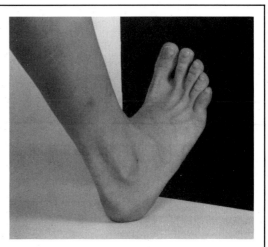

PHASE:
Flexibility

DESCRIPTION:
With the weight on the left foot, place the right foot against a wall. The right heel must be touching the bottom of the pool and the leg should remain straight. Gently press the body forward and hold the stretch for 10 to 60 seconds. Now repeat the same action but with the right knee slightly flexed. Switch legs and repeat.

exercise 85
Knee to Chest

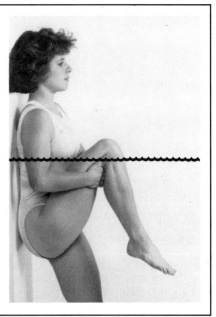

PHASE:
Flexibility

DESCRIPTION:
Stand on the left leg and lean with the back against the pool wall. Flex the right leg and grasp it behind the knee, bringing it up toward the chest. Hold the stretch for 10 to 60 seconds. Switch legs and repeat the exercise.

PRECAUTION:
Keep the knee joint on the weight bearing leg soft.

exercise 86

Hip Flexor Stretch

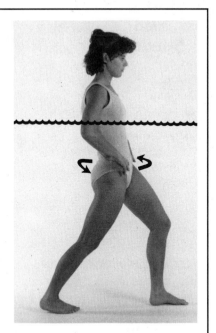

PHASE:
Toning

DESCRIPTION:
Stand in a forward/backward stride position with the knees slightly flexed. Rotate the pelvis backward (the top going backward and the bottom forward). When you feel the tension, hold the stretch for 10 to 60 seconds. Switch the legs and repeat the exercise.

exercise 87
Wall Straddle

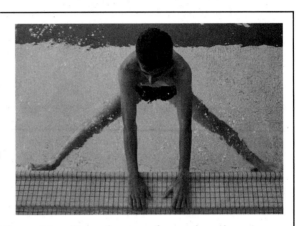

PHASE:
Flexibility

DESCRIPTION:
Hold on to the edge of the pool with the hands and place both feet up against the wall, with the legs in a straddle position. Press the torso forward until tension is felt. Hold for 10 to 60 seconds.

PRECAUTION/MODIFICATION: Keep the knee joints soft. To modify the exercise, lower the legs toward the bottom of the pool.

exercise 88
Tailor

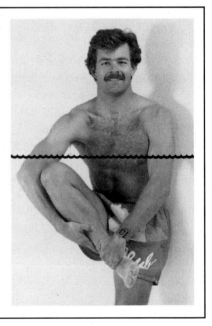

PHASE:
Flexibility

DESCRIPTION:
Stand on the left leg and lean with the back against the pool wall. Place the right elbow against the side of the right knee and grasp the lower leg with the right hand. Now grasp the right ankle with the left hand and pull the foot toward the face. Hold the stretch for 10 to 60 seconds. Switch the position and repeat for the left leg.

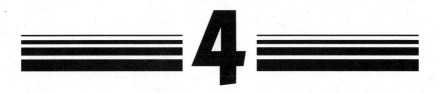

Nutrition
and
Weight Control

The science of nutrition studies the relationship of foods to optimal health and performance. Ample scientific evidence has long linked good nutrition to overall health and well-being. Proper nutrition signifies that a person's diet is supplying all the essential nutrients to carry out normal tissue growth, repair, and maintenance. It also implies that the diet will provide sufficient substrates to obtain the energy necessary for work, physical activity, and relaxation.

Unfortunately, the typical American diet is too high in calories, sugars, fats, sodium, and alcohol; and too low in complex carbohydrates and fiber — none of which are conducive to good health. Over-consumption is now a major concern for many Americans.

The essential nutrients required by the human body are carbohydrates, fats, protein, vitamins, minerals, and water. Carbohydrates, fats, protein, and water are called macronutrients because large amounts are needed on a daily basis. Vitamins and minerals are only necessary in very small amounts, therefore, nutritionists commonly refer to them as micronutrients.

Depending on the amount of nutrients and calories, foods can be categorized into high nutrient density and low nutrient density. High nutrient density is used in reference to foods that contain a low or moderate amount of calories, but are packed with nutrients. Foods that are high in calories but contain few nutrients are of low nutrient density. The latter are frequently referred to as "junk food."

Carbohydrates are the major source of calories used by the body to provide energy for work, cell maintenance, and heat. They also play a crucial role in the digestion and regulation of fat and protein metabolism.

Carbohydrates are divided into simple carbohydrates and complex carbohydrates. Simple carbohydrates (such as candy, pop, and cakes) are frequently denoted as sugars and have little nutritive value. Complex carbohydrates are formed when simple carbohydrates molecules link together. Two examples of complex carbohydrates are starches and dextrins. Starches are commonly found in seeds, corn, nuts, grains, roots, potatoes, and legumes. Dextrins are formed from the breakdown of large starch molecules exposed to dry heat, such as when bread is baked or cold cereals are produced. Complex carbohydrates provide many valuable nutrients to the body and can also be an excellent source of fiber or roughage.

Dietary fiber is a type of complex carbohydrate made up of plant material that cannot be digested by the human body. It is mainly present in leaves, skins, roots, and seeds. Processing and refining foods removes almost all of the natural fiber. In our daily diets, the main sources of dietary fiber are whole-grain cereals and breads, fruits, and vegetables.

Fiber is important in the diet because it may help decrease the risk for cardiovascular disease and cancer. In addition, several other health disorders have been linked to low fiber intake, including constipation, diverticulitis, hemorrhoids, gallbladder disease, and obesity.

Fats or lipids are also used as a source of energy in the human body. They are the most concentrated source of energy. Fats are also a part of the cell structure. They are used as stored energy and as an insulator for body heat preservation. They provide shock absorption, supply essential fatty acids, and carry the fat-soluble vitamins A, D, E, and K.

Proteins are the main substances used to build and repair tissues such as muscles, blood, internal organs, skin, hair, nails, and bones. They are a part of hormones, enzymes, and antibodies and help maintain normal body fluid balance. Proteins can also be used as a source of energy, but only if there are not enough carbohydrates and fats available. The primary sources are meats and alternates, and milk and other dairy products.

Vitamins are organic substances essential for normal metabolism, growth, and development of the body. They are classified into two types based on their solubility: fat-soluble vitamins (A, D, E, and K), and water-soluble vitamins (B complex and C). Vitamins cannot be manufactured by the body; hence, they can only be obtained through a well-balanced diet.

Minerals are inorganic elements found in the body and in food. They serve several important functions. Minerals are constituents of all cells, especially those found in hard parts of the body (bones, nails, teeth). They are crucial in the maintenance of water balance and the acid-base balance. They are essential components of respiratory pigments, enzymes, and enzyme systems, and they regulate muscular and nervous tissue excitability.

Water is the most important nutrient and is involved in almost every vital body process. Approximately 70 percent of total body weight is water. It is used in digestion and absorption of food, in the circulatory process, in removing waste products, in building and rebuilding cells, and in the transport of other nutrients. Water is contained in almost all foods but primarily in liquid foods, fruits, and vegetables. Besides the natural content in foods, it is recommended that every person drink at least eight to ten glasses of fluids a day.

A BALANCED DIET

Most people would like to live life to its fullest, maintain good health, and lead a productive life. One of the fundamental ways to accomplish this goal is by eating a well-balanced diet. Generally, daily caloric intake should be distributed in such a way that 60 percent of the total caloric intake comes from carbohydrates and less than 30 percent from fat. Saturated fats should constitute less than 10 percent of the total daily caloric intake. Protein intake should be about .8 grams per kilogram (2.2 pounds) of body weight. In addition, all of the vitamins, minerals, and water must be provided.

One of the most detrimental health habits facing the American people today is the high amount of fat in the diet. The fat consumption in the average diet is over 40 percent of the total caloric intake. If we want to enjoy better health, a deliberate effort must be made to decrease total fat intake. Therefore, being able to identify sources of fat in the diet is imperative to decrease fat intake.

Each gram of carbohydrates and protein supplies the body with four calories, while fat provides nine calories per gram consumed. In this regard, just looking at the total amount of grams consumed for each type of food can be very misleading. For example, a person who consumes 160 grams of carbohydrates, 100 grams of fat, and 70 grams of protein has a total intake of 330 grams of food. This indicates that 33 percent of the total grams of food are in the form of fat (100 grams of fat ÷ 330 grams of total food × 100). In reality, the diet consists of almost 50 percent fat calories. In this sample diet, 640 calories are derived from carbohydrates (160 grams × 4 calories/gram), 280 calories from protein (70 grams × 4 calories/gram), and 900 calories from fat (100 grams × 9 calories/gram), for a total of 1,820 calories. If 900 calories are derived from fat, you can easily observe that almost half of the total caloric intake is in the form of fat (900 ÷ 1,820 × 100 = 49.5 percent).

Realizing that each gram of fat yields nine calories is a very useful guideline when attempting to determine the fat content of individual foods. All you need to do is multiply the grams of fat by nine and divide by the total calories in that particular food. The percentage is obtained by multiplying the latter figure by 100. For example, if a food label lists a total of 100 calories and 7 grams of fat, the fat content would be 63 percent of total calories. This simple guideline can help you decrease fat intake in your diet.

Achieving and maintaining a balanced diet is not as difficult as most people think. The difficult part is retraining yourself to eat the right type of foods and avoid those that have little or no nutritive value. If you (a) avoid excessive sweets, fats, alcohol, and sodium; (b) increase your fiber intake; and (c) eat the minimum number of servings required for each one of the four basic food groups; you will achieve a well-balanced diet. The minimum number of servings of the four basic food groups for adults are (also see Figure 4.1):

A. Four or more servings per day of beans, grains, and nuts.
B. Four or more servings per day of fruits and vegetables, including one good source of vitamin A (apricots, cantaloupe, broccoli, carrots, pumpkin, and dark leafy vegetables), and one good source of vitamin C (cantaloupe, citrus fruit, kiwi fruit, strawberries, broccoli, cabbage, cauliflower, and green pepper).
C. Two or more servings per day of milk products.
D. Two or more servings per day of poultry, fish, meat and eggs.

Another point of significant interest in nutrition is the unnecessary and sometimes unsafe use of vitamin and mineral supplementation. Even though experts agree that supplements are not necessary, people consume them at a greater rate than ever before. Research has demonstrated that even when a person consumes as few as 1,200 calories per day, no additional supplementation is needed as long as the diet contains the recommended servings from the four basic food groups.

For most people, vitamin and mineral supplementation is unnecessary. Iron deficiency (determined through blood testing) is the only exception for women who suffer from heavy menstrual flow. Pregnant and lactating women may also require supplements. In all instances, supplements should be taken under a physician's supervision. Other people that may benefit from supplementation are alcoholics who are not consuming a balanced diet, strict vegetarians, individuals on extremely low-calorie diets, elderly people who don't regularly receive balanced meals, and newborn infants (usually given a single dose of vitamin K to prevent abnormal bleeding). For healthy people with a balanced diet, supplementation provides no additional health benefits. It will not help a person run faster, jump higher, relieve stress, improve sexual prowess, cure a common cold, or boost energy levels!

Another fallacy regarding nutrition is that many people who regularly eat fast foods high in fat content and/or excessive sweets

Food Group	Recommended Number of Servings				
	Child	Teenager	Adult	Pregnant Woman	Lactating Woman

Milk
1 cup milk, yogurt or
Calcium Equivalent:
  1½ slices (1½ oz.)
    cheddar cheese
  1 cup pudding
  1¾ cups ice cream
  2 cups cottage cheese*
	3	4	2	4	4

Meat
2 ounces cooked, lean meat,
fish, poultry, or
Protein Equivalent:
  2 eggs
  2 slices (2 oz.) cheddar
    cheese*
  ½ cup cottage cheese*
  1 cup dried beans, peas
  4 tbsp. peanut butter
	2	2	2	3	2

Fruit–Vegetable
  ½ cup cooked or juice
  1 cup raw
  Portion commonly served
  such as a medium-size
  apple or banana
	4	4	4	4	4

Grain, whole grain,
fortified, enriched
  1 slice bread
  1 cup ready-to-eat cereal
  ½ cup cooked cereal,
    pasta, grits
	4	4	4	4	4

*Count cheese as serving of milk OR meat, not both simultaneously.

"Others" complement but do not replace foods from the Four Food Groups. Amounts should be determined by individual caloric needs.

FIGURE 4.1. Recommended Number of Servings from the Four Basic Food Groups.

feel that vitamin and mineral supplementation is needed to balance their diet. The problem in these cases is not a lack of vitamins and minerals, but rather that the diet is too high in calories, fat, and sodium. Supplementation will not offset such poor eating habits.

▬ EATING DISORDERS

Anorexia nervosa and bulimia have been classified as physical and emotional problems usually developed as a result of individual, family, and/or social pressures to achieve thinness. These medical disorders are steadily increasing in most industrialized nations, where low-calorie diets and model-like thinness are normal behaviors encouraged by society. Individuals who suffer from eating disorders have an intense fear of becoming obese, which does not disappear even as extreme amounts of weight are lost.

Anorexia nervosa is a condition of self-imposed starvation to lose and then maintain very low body weight. The anorexic seems to fear weight gain more than death from starvation. Furthermore, these individuals have a distorted image of their body and perceive themselves as being fat even when critically emaciated.

Although a genetic predisposition may exist, the anorexic patient often comes from a mother-dominated home, with other possible drug addictions in the family. The syndrome may start following a stressful life event and the uncertainty of the ability to cope efficiently. Because the female role in society is changing more rapidly, women seem to be especially susceptible. Life events such as weight gain, start of menstrual periods, beginning of college, loss of a boyfriend, poor self-esteem, social rejection, start of a professional career, and/or becoming a wife or mother may trigger the syndrome. The person usually begins a diet and may initially feel in control and happy about weight loss, even if not overweight.

To speed up the weight loss process, severe dieting is frequently combined with exhaustive exercise and overuse of laxatives and/or diuretics. The individual commonly develops obsessive and compulsive behaviors and emphatically denies the condition. There also appears to be a constant preoccupation with food, meal planning, grocery shopping, and unusual eating habits.

As weight is lost and health begins to deteriorate, the anorexic feels weak and tired and may realize that there is a problem but will not discontinue starvation and refuses to accept the behavior as abnormal.

Once significant weight loss and malnutrition begin, typical physical changes become more visible. Some of the more common changes exhibited by anorexics are amenorrhea (cessation of menstruation), digestive difficulties, extreme sensitivity to cold, hair and skin problems, fluid and electrolyte abnormalities (which may lead to an irregular heartbeat and sudden stopping of the heart), injuries to nerves and tendons, abnormalities of immune function, anemia, growth of fine body hair, mental confusion, inability to concentrate, lethargy, depression, skin dryness, and decreased skin and body temperature.

Many of the changes of anorexia nervosa are by no means irreversible. Treatment almost always requires professional help and the sooner it is started, the higher the chances for reversibility and cure. A combination of medical and psychological techniques are used in therapy to restore proper nutrition, prevent medical complications, and modify the environment or events that triggered the syndrome. Seldom are anorexics able to overcome the problem by themselves.

Unfortunately, there is strong denial among anorexics and they are able to hide their condition and deceive friends and relatives quite effectively. Based on their behavior, many individuals meet all of the characteristics of anorexia nervosa, but the condition goes undetected because both thinness and dieting are socially acceptable behaviors. Only a well-trained clinician is able to make a positive diagnosis.

Bulimia, a pattern of binge eating and purging, is more prevalent than anorexia nervosa. For many years it was thought to be a variant of anorexia nervosa, but it is now identified as a separate disease.

Bulimics are usually healthy-looking people, well educated, near ideal body weight, who enjoy food and often socialize around it. However, they are emotionally insecure, rely on others, and lack self-confidence and esteem. Maintenance of ideal weight and food are both important to them. As a result of stressful life events or simple compulsion to eat, they periodically engage in binge eating that may last an hour or longer, during which several thousand calories may be consumed. A feeling of deep guilt and shame then follows, along with intense fear of gaining weight. Purging seems to be an easy answer to the problem, and the binging cycle continues without the fear of gaining weight. The most common form of purging is self-induced vomiting, although strong laxatives and emetics are frequently used. Near-fasting diets and strenuous bouts of physical activity are also commonly seen in bulimics.

Medical problems associated with bulimia include cardiac arrhythmias, amenorrhea, kidney and bladder damage, ulcers, colitis, tearing of the esophagus and/or stomach, teeth erosion, gum damage, and general muscular weakness.

Unlike anorexics, bulimics realize that their behavior is abnormal and feel great shame for their actions. Fearing social rejection, the binge-purging cycle is primarily carried out in secrecy and during unusual hours of the day. Nevertheless, bulimia can be treated successfully when the person realizes that such destructive behavior is not the solution to life's problems. Hopefully, the change in attitude will grasp the individual before permanent or fatal damage is done.

PRINCIPLES OF WEIGHT CONTROL

Achieving and maintaining ideal body weight is a major objective of a good physical fitness program. Estimates, however, indicate that only about 10 percent of all people who ever initiate a traditional weight loss program are able to lose the desired weight, and worse yet, only one in 100 is able to keep the weight off for a significant period of time. You may ask why the traditional diets have failed. The answer is simply because very few diets teach the importance of lifetime changes in food selection and the role of exercise as the keys to successful weight loss.

There are several reasons why fad diets continue to deceive people and can claim that weight will indeed be lost if "all" instructions are followed. Most diets are very low in calories and/or deprive the body of certain nutrients, creating a metabolic imbalance that can even cause death. Under such conditions, a lot of the weight loss is in the form of water and protein and not fat. On a crash diet, close to 50 percent of the weight loss is in lean (protein) tissue. When the body uses protein instead of a combination of fats and carbohydrates as a source of energy, weight is lost as much as ten times faster. A gram of protein yields half the amount of energy that fat does. In the case of muscle protein, one-fifth of protein is mixed with four-fifths water. In other words, each pound of muscle yields only one-tenth the amount of energy of a pound of fat. As a result, most of the weight loss is in the form of water, which on the scale, of course, looks good. Nevertheless, when regular eating habits are resumed, most of the lost weight comes right back.

Some diets only allow the consumption of certain foods. If people would only realize that there are no "magic" foods that will provide all the necessary nutrients and that a person has to eat a variety of foods to be well nourished, the diet industry would not be as successful. The unfortunate thing about most of these diets is that they create a nutritional deficiency which at times can be fatal. The reason why some of these diets succeed is because in due time people get tired of eating the same thing day in and day out and eventually start eating less. If they happen to achieve the lower weight, once they go back to old eating habits without implementing permanent dietary changes, weight is quickly gained back again.

A few diets recommend exercise along with caloric restrictions, which, of course, is the best method for weight reduction. A lot of the weight lost is due to exercise; hence, the diet has achieved its purpose. Unfortunately, if no permanent changes in food selection and activity level take place, once dieting and exercise are discontinued, the weight is quickly gained back.

Even though only a few years ago the principles that govern a weight loss and maintenance program seemed to be pretty clear, we now know that the final answers are not yet in. The traditional concepts related to weight control have been centered around three assumptions: (1) that balancing food intake against output allows a person to achieve ideal weight, (2) that fat people just eat too much, and (3) that it really does not matter to the human body how much (or little) fat is stored. While there may be some truth to these statements, they are still open to much debate and research.

Every person has a certain amount of body fat which is regulated by genetic and environmental factors. The genetic instinct to survive tells the body that fat storage is vital, and therefore it sets an inherently acceptable fat level. This level remains pretty constant or may gradually climb due to poor lifestyle habits. For instance, under strict caloric reductions, the body may make extreme metabolic adjustments in an effort to maintain its fat storage. The basal metabolic rate may drop dramatically against a consistent negative caloric balance (as in dieting), and a person may be on a plateau for days or even weeks without losing much weight. When the dieter goes back to the normal or even below normal caloric intake, at which the weight may have been stable for a long period of time, the fat loss is quickly regained as the body strives to regain a comfortable fat store.

Let's use a practical illustration. A person would like to lose some body fat and assumes that a stable body weight has been reached at an average daily caloric intake of 1,800 calories (no weight gain or loss occurs at this daily intake). This person now starts a strict low-calorie diet, or even worse, a near-fasting diet in an attempt to achieve rapid weight loss. Immediately the body activates its survival mechanism and readjusts its metabolism to a lower caloric balance. After a few weeks of dieting at less than 400 to 600 calories per day, the body can now maintain its normal functions at 1,000 calories per day. Having lost the desired weight, the person terminates the diet but realizes that the original caloric intake of 1,800 calories per day will need to be decreased to maintain the new lower weight. Therefore, to adjust to the new lower body weight, the intake is restricted to about 1,500 calories per day, but the individual is surprised to find that even at this lower daily intake (300 fewer calories), weight is gained back at a rate of one pound every one to two weeks. This new lowered metabolic rate may take a year or more after terminating the diet to kick back up to its normal level.

From this explanation, it is clear that individuals should never go on very low-calorie diets. Not only will this practice decrease resting metabolic rate, but it will also deprive the body of the basic daily nutrients required for normal physiological functions. Under no circumstances should a person ever engage in diets below 1,200 and 1,500 calories for women and men, respectively. Remember that weight (fat) is gained over a period of months and years and not overnight. Equally, weight loss should be accomplished gradually and not abruptly. Daily caloric intakes of 1,200 to 1,500

calories will still provide the necessary nutrients if properly distributed over the four basic food groups (meeting the daily required
servings from each group). Of course, the individual will have to
learn which foods meet the requirements and yet are low in fat,
sugar, and calories.

Furthermore, when weight loss is pursued by means of dietary
restrictions alone, there will always be a decrease in lean body
mass (muscle protein, along with vital organ protein). The
amount of lean body mass lost depends exclusively on the caloric
restriction of your diet. In near-fasting diets, up to 50 percent of
the weight loss can be lean body mass, and the other 50 percent
will be actual fat loss. When diet is combined with exercise, 98 percent of the weight loss will be in the form of fat, and there may
actually be an increase in lean tissue. Lean body mass loss is never
desirable because it weakens the organs and muscles and slows
down the metabolism.

Decreases in lean body mass are commonly seen in severely
restricted diets. There are no diets with caloric intakes below 1,200
to 1,500 calories that can insure no loss of lean body mass. Even
at this intake, there is some loss unless the diet is combined with
exercise. Many diets have claimed that the lean component is unal-
tered with their particular diet, but the simple truth is that regardless of what nutrients may be added to the diet, if caloric restrictions are too severe, there will always be a loss of lean tissue.

Unfortunately, too many people constantly engage in low-
calorie diets, and every time they do so, the metabolic rate keeps
slowing down as more lean tissue is lost. It is not uncommon to
find individuals in their forties or older who weigh the same as
they did when they were twenty and feel that they are at ideal
body weight. Nevertheless, during this span of twenty years or
more, they have "dieted" all too many times without engaging in
physical activity. The weight is regained shortly after terminating
each diet, but most of that gain is in fat. Perhaps at age twenty
they weighed 150 pounds and were only 15 to 16 percent fat. Now
at age forty, even though they still weigh 150 pounds, they may
be 30 to 40 percent fat. They may feel that they are at ideal body
weight and wonder why they are eating very little and still have
a difficult time maintaining that weight.

Research has also shown that a diet high in fats and refined
carbohydrates, near-fasting diets, and perhaps even artificial

sweeteners will not allow a person to lose weight; and on the contrary only contribute to weight (fat) gain. Therefore, it looks as though the only practical and effective way to lose fat weight is through a combination of exercise and a diet high in complex carbohydrates and low in fat and sugar.

Because of the effects of proper food management, many nutritionists now believe that the total number of calories should not be a concern in a weight control program, but rather the source of those calories. In this regard, most of the effort is spent in retraining eating habits, increasing the intake of complex carbohydrates and high-fiber foods, and decreasing the use of refined carbohydrates (sugars) and fats. In addition, a "diet" is no longer viewed as a temporary tool to aid in weight loss, but rather as a permanent change in eating behaviors to insure adequate weight management and health enhancement. The role of increased physical activity must also be considered, because successful weight loss, maintenance, and ideal body composition are seldom achieved without a regular exercise program.

Exercise: The Key to Successful Weight Management

Perhaps the most significant factor in achieving ideal body composition is a lifetime exercise program. For individuals who are trying to lose weight, a combination of an aerobic and some type of strength-training program works best. Because of the continuity and duration of aerobic activities, large numbers of calories are burned during a single bout of exercise (about 400 to 600 per hour).

Strength-training exercises have the greatest impact in increasing lean body mass. Each additional pound of muscle tissue can raise the basal metabolic rate between 50 and 100 calories per day. Using the conservative estimate of 50 calories per day, an individual who adds five pounds of muscle tissue as a result of strength training would increase the basal metabolic rate by 250 calories per day, or the equivalent of 91,250 calories per year.

Since exercise leads to an increase in lean body mass, it is not uncommon for body weight to remain the same or increase when you initiate an exercise program, while inches and percent body fat decrease. The increase in lean tissue results in an increased functional capacity of the human body. With exercise, most of the weight loss is seen after a few weeks of training — when the lean component has stabilized.

It is also important to clarify that there is no such thing as spot reducing or losing "cellulite" from certain body parts. Cellulite is nothing but plain fat storage. Just doing several sets of daily sit-ups will not help to get rid of fat in the midsection of the body. When fat comes off, it does so from throughout the entire body, and not just the exercised area. The greatest proportion of fat may come off the largest fat deposits, but the caloric output of a few sets of sit-ups is practically nil and does not have a real effect on total body fat reduction. The amount of exercise has to be much longer to have a real impact on weight reduction.

Dieting has never been fun and never will be. Individuals who have a weight problem and are serious about losing weight will have to make exercise a regular part of their daily life, along with proper food management, and perhaps even sensible adjustments in caloric intake.

Significantly overweight individuals may also have to choose activities where they will not have to support their own body weight, but that will still be effective in burning calories. Joint and muscle injuries are very common among overweight individuals who participate in weight-bearing exercises such as walking, jogging, and aerobic dancing. Some better alternatives are water aerobics, walking in a shallow pool, running in place in deep water (treading water), or riding a bicycle (either road or stationary). Water aerobics is quickly gaining popularity and seems to be just as effective as other forms of aerobic activity in helping individuals lose weight without the "pain" and fear of injuries.

One final benefit of exercise related to weight control is that fat can be burned more efficiently. Since both carbohydrates and fats are sources of energy, when the glucose levels begin to decrease during prolonged exercise, more fat is used as energy substrate. Equally important is the fact that fat-burning enzymes increase with aerobic training. The role of these enzymes is significant, because fat can only be lost by burning it in muscle. As the concentration of the enzymes increases, so does the ability to burn fat.

The time of day when food is consumed may also play a role in weight reduction. A study conducted at the Aerobics Research Center in Dallas, Texas, indicated that when on a diet, weight is lost most effectively if the majority of the calories are consumed before 1:00 p.m. and not during the evening meal. The recommendation made at this center is that when a person is attempting to lose weight, a minimum of 25 percent of the total daily calories should be consumed for breakfast, 50 percent for lunch, and 25 percent or less at dinner. Other experts have indicated that if most of your daily calories are consumed during one meal, the body may perceive that something is wrong and will slow down your metabolism so that it can store a greater amount of calories in the form of fat. Also, eating most of the calories in one meal causes you to go hungry the rest of the day, making it more difficult to adhere to the diet.

▬ TIPS TO HELP CHANGE BEHAVIOR AND ADHERE ▬ TO A LIFETIME WEIGHT MANAGEMENT PROGRAM

Achieving and maintaining ideal body composition is by no means an impossible task, but it does require desire and commitment. If adequate weight management is to become a priority in life, people must realize that some retraining of behavior is crucial for success. Modifying old habits and developing new positive behaviors take time. The following list of management techniques has been successfully used by individuals to change detrimental behavior and adhere to a positive lifetime weight control program. People are not expected to use all of the strategies listed, but they should check the ones that would apply and help them in developing a retraining program.

1. **Commitment to change.** The first ingredient to modify behavior is the desire to do so. The reasons for change must be more important than those for carrying on with present lifestyle patterns. People must accept the fact that there is a problem and decide by themselves whether they really want to change. If a sincere commitment is there, the chances for success are already enhanced.

2. **Set realistic goals.** Most people with a weight problem would like to lose weight in a relatively short period of time but fail to realize that the weight problem developed over a span of several years. In setting a realistic long-term

goal, short-term objectives should also be planned. The long-term goal may be a decrease in body fat to 20 percent of total body weight. The short-term objective may be a 1 percent decrease in body fat each month. Such objectives allow for regular evaluation and help maintain motivation and renewed commitment to achieve the long-term goal.

3. **Incorporate exercise into the program.** Selecting enjoyable activities, places, times, equipment, and people to work with enhances exercise adherence. Details on developing a complete exercise program are found in Chapter 3.

4. **Develop healthy eating patterns.** Plan on eating three regular meals per day consistent with the body's nutritional requirements. Learn to differentiate between hunger and appetite. Hunger is the actual physical need for food. Appetite is a desire for food, usually triggered by factors such as stress, habit, boredom, depression, food availability, or just the thought of food itself. Eating only when there is a physical need is wise weight management. In this regard, developing and sticking to a regular meal pattern helps control hunger.

5. **Avoid automatic eating.** Many people associate certain daily activities with eating. For example, people eat while cooking, watching television, reading, talking on the telephone, or visiting with neighbors. Most of the time, the foods consumed in such situations lack nutritional value or are high in sugar and fat.

6. **Stay busy.** People tend to eat more when they sit around and do nothing. Keeping the mind and body occupied with activities not associated with eating helps decrease the desire to eat. Try walking, cycling, playing sports, gardening, sewing, or visiting a library, a museum, a park, etc. Develop other skills and interests or try something new and exciting to break the routine of life.

7. **Plan your meals ahead of time.** Wise shopping is required to accomplish this objective (by the way, when shopping, do so on a full stomach, since such a practice

will decrease impulsive buying of unhealthy foods — and then snacking on the way home). Include whole-grain breads and cereals, fruits and vegetables, low-fat milk and dairy products, lean meats, fish, and poultry.

8. **Cook wisely.** Decrease the use of fat and refined foods in food preparation. Trim all visible fat off meats and remove skin off poultry prior to cooking. Skim the fat off gravies and soups. Bake, broil, and boil instead of frying. Use butter, cream, mayonnaise, and salad dressings sparingly. Avoid shellfish, coconut oil, palm oil, and cocoa butter. Prepare plenty of bulky foods. Add whole-grain breads and cereals, vegetables, and legumes to most meals. Try fruits for dessert. Beware of soda pop, fruit juices, and fruit-flavored drinks (these beverages are usually high in sugar). Drink plenty of water — at least six glasses a day.

9. **Do not serve more food than can or should be eaten.** Measure the food portions and keep serving dishes away from the table. In this manner, less food is consumed, seconds are more difficult to obtain, and appetite is decreased because food is not visible. People should not be forced to eat when they are satisfied (including children after they have already had a healthy, nutritious serving).

10. **Learn to eat slowly and at the table only.** Eating is one of the pleasures of life, and we need to take time to enjoy it. Eating on the run is detrimental because the body is not given sufficient time to "register" nutritive and caloric consumption, and overeating usually occurs before the fullness signal is perceived. Always eating at the table also forces people to take time out to eat and will decrease snacking between meals, primarily because of the extra time and effort that are required to sit down and eat. When done eating, do not sit around the table. Clean up and put the food away to avoid unnecessary snacking.

11. **Avoid social binges.** Social gatherings are a common place for self-defeating behavior. Do not feel pressured to eat or drink, nor rationalize in these situations. Choose low-calorie foods and entertain yourself with other activities such as dancing and talking.

12. **Beware of raids on the refrigerator and the cookie jar.** When such occur, attempt to take control of the situation. Stop and think what is taking place. For those who have difficulty in avoiding such raids, environmental management is recommended. Do not bring high-calorie, high-sugar, and/or high-fat foods into the house. If they are brought into the house, they ought to be stored in places where they are difficult to get to or are less visible. If they are unseen or not readily available, there will be less temptation. Keeping them in places like the garage and basement may be sufficient to discourage many people from taking the time and effort to go get them. By no means should treats be completely eliminated, but all things should be done in moderation.

13. **Practice adequate stress management techniques.** Many people snack and increase food consumption when confronted with stressful situations. Eating is not a stress-releasing activity and can in reality aggravate the problem if weight control is an issue.

14. **Monitor changes and reward accomplishments.** Feedback on fat loss, lean tissue gain, and/or weight loss is a reward in itself. Awareness of changes in body composition also helps reinforce new behaviors. Furthermore, being able to exercise uninterruptedly for 15, 20, 30, 60 minutes, or swimming a certain distance, running a mile, etc., are all accomplishments that deserve recognition. When certain objectives are met, rewards that are not related to eating are encouraged. Buy new clothing, a tennis racket, a bicycle, exercise shoes, or something else that is special and would have not been acquired otherwise.

15. **Think positive.** Avoid negative thoughts on how difficult it might be to change past behaviors. Instead, think of the benefits that will be reaped, such as feeling, looking, and functioning better, plus enjoying better health and improving the quality of life. Attempt to stay away from negative environments and people who will not be supportive. Those who do not have the same desires and/or encourage self-defeating behaviors should be avoided.

IN CONCLUSION

There is no simple and quick way to take off excessive body fat and keep it off for good. Weight management is accomplished through a lifetime commitment to physical activity and adequate food selection. When engaged in a weight (fat) reduction program, people may also have to moderately decrease caloric intake and implement appropriate strategies to modify unhealthy eating behaviors.

During the process of behavior modification, it is almost inevitable to relapse and engage in past negative behaviors. Nevertheless, making mistakes is human and does not necessarily mean failure. Failure comes to those who give up and do not use previous experiences to build upon and, in turn, develop appropriate skills that will prevent self-defeating behaviors in the future. "If there is a will, there is a way," and those who persist will reap the rewards.

5

A Healthy
Lifestyle Approach

Although most individuals in the United States are firm believers in the benefits of physical activity and positive lifestyle habits as a means to promote better health, most do not reap these benefits because they simply do not know how to implement a healthy lifestyle program that will indeed yield the desired results. Unfortunately, many of the present lifestyle patterns of the American people are such a serious threat to our health that they actually increase the deterioration rate of the human body and often lead to premature illness and mortality.

Scientific evidence has clearly shown that improving the quality and most likely the longevity of our lives is a matter of personal choice. Therefore, in addition to the information already presented in the first four chapters of this book, the materials presented in this last chapter have been written to complement your water aerobics fitness program with a comprehensive healthy lifestyle program. This combination of fitness with an overall healthy lifestyle program has been referred to by the experts as the wellness approach to better health and quality of life.

Wellness has been defined as the constant and deliberate effort to stay healthy and achieve the highest potential for total well-being.

The concept of wellness incorporates many other components other than those associated with physical fitness, such as proper nutrition, cardiovascular risk reduction, cancer prevention, smoking cessation, stress management, substance abuse control, and health education (see Figure 5.1).

The difference between physical fitness and wellness is best illustrated in the following example. An individual who is running three miles per day, lifting weights regularly, participating in stretching exercises, and maintaining ideal body weight, can easily be classified in the good or excellent category for each one of the fitness components. However, if this person suffers from high blood pressure, smokes, consumes alcohol, and/or eats a diet high in fatty foods, the individual is probably developing several risk factors for cardiovascular disease and cancer and may not be aware of it. A risk factor is defined as an asymptomatic state that a person has that may lead to disease. Consequently, the biggest challenge we are faced with today is to teach individuals how to take control of their personal health habits to insure a better, healthier, happier, and more productive life.

Based on current statistical estimates, the leading causes of death in the country today are basically lifestyle related. About 70 percent of all deaths are caused by cardiovascular disease (includes heart disease and cerebro-vascular diseases) and cancer. Approximately 80 percent of these could be prevented through a positive lifestyle program. Accidents are the third cause of death. While not all accidents are preventable, many are. A significant amount of fatal accidents are related to alcohol and lack of use of seat belts. The fourth cause of death, chronic obstructive pulmonary disease, is largely related to tobacco use.

▬ CARDIOVASCULAR DISEASE

The most prevalent degenerative diseases in the United States are those of the cardiovascular system. Close to one-half of all deaths in the country result from cardiovascular disease. The disease refers to any pathological condition that affects the heart and the circulatory system (blood vessels). Some examples of cardiovascular diseases are coronary heart disease, peripheral vascular disease, congenital heart disease, rheumatic heart disease,

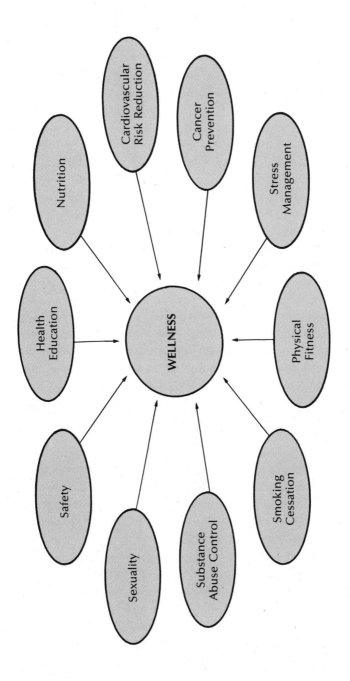

FIGURE 5.1. Wellness Components

atherosclerosis, strokes, high blood pressure, and congestive heart failure.

According to the American Heart Association, heart and blood vessel disease costs were in excess of $83.7 billion in 1985. Heart attacks alone cost American industry 132 million workdays annually, including $12.4 billion in lost productivity because of physical and emotional disability.

It must also be noted that in the case of coronary heart disease, about 50 percent of the time the first symptom of this disease is a heart attack itself. Forty percent of the people who suffer a first heart attack die within the first 24 hours. In one out of every five cardiovascular deaths, sudden death is the initial symptom. Close to 200,000 of those that die are people in their most productive years between the ages of 30 and 65.

Additionally, the American Heart Association estimates that over $700 million a year are spent in replacing employees who are recovering from heart attacks. Oddly enough, most coronary heart disease risk factors are reversible and can be controlled by the individuals themselves through appropriate lifestyle modifications.

Even though cardiovascular disease is still the leading cause of death in the country, the mortality rates for this disease have been decreasing in the last two decades. In the last few years, approximately 200,000 people were saved each year that were expected to die as a direct result of heart and blood vessel disease. This reduction is attributed primarily to prevention programs dealing with risk factor management and to better health care.

The major form of cardiovascular disease is coronary heart disease (CHD), a condition in which the arteries that supply the heart muscle with oxygen and nutrients are narrowed by fatty deposits such as cholesterol and triglycerides. The narrowing of the coronary arteries diminishes the blood supply to the heart muscle, which can eventually lead to a heart attack. CHD is the single leading cause of death in the United States, accounting for approximately one-third of all deaths and more than half of all cardiovascular deaths.

The leading risk factors that contribute to the development of CHD have been identified and are discussed in this chapter. An important concept in CHD risk management is that with the exception of age, family history of heart disease, and certain electrocardiogram abnormalities, all of the other risk factors are preventable and reversible, and risk reduction can be accomplished by the individual. To aid in the implementation of a lifetime risk reduction program, the following guidelines should be implemented:

1. **Cardiovascular endurance.** Improving cardiovascular endurance through aerobic exercise has perhaps the greatest impact in overall heart disease risk reduction. In this regard, you need to be sure to engage in a lifetime aerobic exercise program, training a minimum of three times per week, in the appropriate target zone, for about 20 to 30 minutes per workout. In the words of Dr. Kenneth H. Cooper, pioneer of the aerobic movement in the United States, the evidence of the benefits of aerobic exercise in the reduction of heart disease is "far too impressive to be ignored."

2. **Blood pressure.** Blood pressure should be checked regularly, regardless of whether elevation is present or not. Ideal blood pressure should be 120/80 or below. The American Heart Association considers all blood pressures over 140/90 as hypertension. Regular physical exercise, weight control, a low-salt diet, smoking cessation, and stress management are the basic guidelines for blood pressure control.

3. **Body composition.** Maintenance of recommended body weight (fat percent) is essential in any cardiovascular risk reduction program.

4. **Blood lipid profile.** The term "blood lipids" (fats) is mainly used in reference to cholesterol and triglycerides. If you have never had a blood lipid test, it is highly recommended that you have one in the near future. Your blood test should include total cholesterol, HDL-cholesterol (high density lipoprotein cholesterol), and triglycerides. A significant elevation in blood lipids has long been clearly linked to heart and blood vessel disease.

   Only a few years ago the general recommendation was to keep total blood cholesterol levels below 200 mg/dl (milligrams per deciliter). For individuals thirty and younger it is now recommended that the total cholesterol count should not exceed 180 mg/dl. Even though these guidelines should still be followed, the crucial factor seems to be the way in which cholesterol is "packaged" or carried in the bloodstream rather than the total amount present.

Cholesterol is primarily transported or packaged in the form of high-density lipoprotein cholesterol (HDL-cholesterol) and low-density lipoprotein cholesterol (LDL-cholesterol). The high-density molecules have a high affinity for cholesterol and tend to attract cholesterol, which is then carried to the liver to be metabolized and excreted. In other words, they act as "scavengers" removing cholesterol from the body, thus preventing plaque formation in the arteries. On the other hand, LDL-cholesterol tends to release cholesterol, which may then penetrate the lining of the arteries, enhancing the process of atherosclerosis.

From the previous discussion, it can easily be seen that the more HDL-cholesterol present, the better. HDL-cholesterol is the so called "good cholesterol" and offers a certain degree of protection against heart disease. Many authorities now believe that the ratio of total cholesterol to HDL-cholesterol is a better indicator of potential risk for cardiovascular disease than the total value by itself. It is generally accepted that a 4.5 or lower ratio (total cholesterol/HDL-cholesterol) is excellent for men, and 4.0 or lower is best for women. For instance, 50 mg/dl of HDL-cholesterol as compared to 200 mg/dl of total cholesterol yields a ratio of 4.0 (200 ÷ 50 = 4.0). Furthermore, HDL-cholesterol levels in the high 40s (or higher) seem to offer the best protection.

As a general rule of thumb, the following dietary guidelines are recommended to lower LDL-cholesterol levels: (a) egg consumption should be limited to less than three eggs per week; (b) red meats should be eaten less than three times per week, and organ meats (e.g., liver and kidneys), sausage, bacon, hot dogs, and canned meats should be avoided; (c) low-fat milk (1 percent or less preferably) and low-fat dairy products are recommended; (d) shellfish, coconut oil, palm oil, and cocoa butter should be avoided or used sparingly; and (e) ideal body weight should be achieved. Aerobic exercise is also crucial, because it helps increase HDL-cholesterol.

Triglycerides are carried in the bloodstream primarily by very low-density lipoproteins (VLDL) and chylomicrons. These fatty acids are found in poultry skin, lunch meats, and shellfish. However, they are mainly manufactured in the liver from refined sugars, starches, and alcohol. High intake of alcohol and sugars (honey included) will significantly increase triglyceride levels. Thus, they can be lowered by decreasing the consumption of the above-mentioned foods along with weight reduction (if overweight) and aerobic exercise. An optimal blood triglyceride level is less than 100 mg/dl.

5. **Stress electrocardiogram (ECG).** A stress ECG is also known as a maximal exercise tolerance test. Similar to a high-speed road test on a car, a stress ECG reveals the tolerance of the heart to high-intensity exercise. It is frequently used to diagnose coronary heart disease. It is also used to determine cardiovascular fitness levels, to screen persons for preventive and cardiac rehabilitation programs, to detect abnormal blood pressure response during exercise, and to establish actual or functional maximal heart rate for exercise prescription purposes.

While not every adult who wishes to start an exercise program needs a stress ECG, the following guidelines can be used to determine when this type of test should be administered:

- Adults forty-five years or older.

- A total cholesterol level above 200 mg/dl, or a total cholesterol/HDL-cholesterol ratio above 4.0 for women and 4.5 for men.

- Hypertensive and diabetic patients.

- Cigarette smokers.

- Individuals with a family history of coronary heart disease, syncope, or sudden death before age sixty.

- All individuals with symptoms of chest discomfort, dysrhythmias, syncope, or chronotropic incompetence (a heart rate that increases slowly during exercise and never reaches maximum).

6. **Smoking.** Cigarette smoking is the single largest preventable cause of illness and premature death in the United States. When considering all related deaths, smoking is responsible for approximately 250,000 unnecessary deaths each year. There is a definite increase in death rates from heart disease, cancer, stroke, aortic aneurysm, chronic bronchitis, emphysema, and peptic ulcers.

   In relation to cardiovascular disease, cigarette smoking not only speeds up the process of atherosclerosis (fatty buildup on the walls of the arteries), but there is also a threefold increase in the risk of sudden death following a myocardial infarction. Smoking increases heart rate, blood pressure, and the irritability of the heart, which can trigger fatal cardiac arrhythmias. Experts have indicated that as far as the extra load on the heart is concerned, giving up one pack of cigarettes per day is the equivalent of losing between fifty and seventy-five pounds of excess body fat! Another harmful effect is a decrease in HDL-cholesterol, or the "good type" that helps control your blood lipids.

   Pipe and/or cigar smoking and chewing tobacco also increase risk for heart disease. Even if no smoke is inhaled, certain amounts of toxic substances can be absorbed through the mouth membranes and end up in the bloodstream. Individuals who use tobacco in any of these three forms also have a much greater risk for cancer of the oral cavity.

   Cigarette smoking, along with a poor total cholesterol/HDL-cholesterol ratio and high blood pressure, are the three most significant risk factors for coronary disease. Nevertheless, the risk for both cardiovascular disease and cancer starts to decrease the moment you quit. The risk approaches that of a lifetime nonsmoker ten and fifteen years, respectively, following cessation.

7. **Tension and stress.** Tension and stress have become a normal part of every person's life. Everyone has to deal with goals, deadlines, responsibilities, pressures, etc., in daily life. Almost everything in life (whether positive or negative) is a source of stress. However, it is not the stressor itself that creates the health hazard, but rather the

individual's response to it that may pose a health problem. Individuals who are under a lot of stress and cannot relax will experience a constant low-level strain on the cardiovascular system that could manifest itself in the form of heart disease.

Physical exercise has been found to be one of the best ways to relieve stress. When an individual engages in physical activity, stress is dissipated and consequently the person is able to relax. Exercise also increases muscular activity, which causes muscular relaxation upon completion of physical activity.

8. **Personal and family history.** Individuals who have a family history or have already suffered from cardiovascular problems are at higher risk than those who have never had a problem. People with such a history should be strongly encouraged to maintain the other risk factors as low as possible. Since most risk factors are reversible, this practice significantly decreases the risk for future problems.

9. **Age.** Age is a risk factor because of the greater incidence of heart disease among older people. This tendency may be partly induced by an increased risk among the other factors due to changes in lifestyle as we get older (less physical activity, poor nutrition, obesity, etc.).

Young people, however, should not feel that heart disease will not affect them. The disease process begins early in life. Autopsies conducted on young people who died in their twenties have revealed early stages of atherosclerosis. Other studies have found elevated blood cholesterol levels in children as young as ten years old.

While the aging process cannot be stopped, it can certainly be slowed down. It has often been said that certain individuals in their sixties or older possess the bodies of twenty-year-olds. The opposite also holds true: twenty-year-olds often are in such poor condition and health that they almost seem to have the bodies of sixty-year-olds. Adequate risk factor management and positive lifestyle habits are the best ways to slow down the natural aging process.

CANCER

Cancer is defined as an uncontrolled growth and spread of abnormal cells in the body. Some cells grow into a mass of tissue called a tumor, which can be either benign or malignant. A malignant tumor would be considered a "cancer". If the spread of cells is not controlled, death ensues. Over 22 percent of all deaths in the United States are due to cancer. About 494,000 people died of this disease in 1988, and an estimated 985,000 new cases were expected the same year.

As with cardiovascular disease, cancer is largely a preventable disease. The biggest factor in fighting cancer today is health education. As much as 80 percent of all human cancers are related to lifestyle or environmental factors (includes diet, tobacco use, excessive use of alcohol, overexposure to sunlight, and exposure to occupational hazards). Most of these cancers could be prevented through positive lifestyle habits.

Equally important is the fact that cancer is now viewed as the most curable of all chronic diseases. Over half of all cancers are curable. Over five million Americans were alive in 1988 who had a history of cancer. Close to three million of them were considered cured.

The most effective way to protect against cancer is by changing negative lifestyle habits and behaviors that have been practiced for years. The American Cancer Society has issued the following recommendations in regard to cancer prevention:

1. **Dietary changes.** The diet should be low in fat and high in fiber, with ample amounts of vitamins A and C from natural sources. Cruciferous vegetables are encouraged in the diet, alcohol should be used in moderation, and obesity should be avoided.

   High fat intake has been linked primarily to breast, colon, and prostate cancers. Low fiber intake seems to increase the risk of colon cancer. Foods high in vitamins A and C may help decrease the incidence of larynx, esophagus, and lung cancers. Additionally, salt-cured, smoked, and nitrite-cured foods should be avoided. These foods have been linked to cancer of the esophagus and stomach. Vitamin C seems to help decrease the formation of nitrosamines (cancer-causing substances that are formed when cured meats are eaten). Cruciferous vegetables (cauliflower, broccoli, Brussels sprouts, and kohlrabi) should be included in the diet, since they seem to decrease the risk for the development of certain cancers.

Alcohol should be used in moderation. Alcoholism increases the risk of certain cancers, especially when combined with tobacco smoking or smokeless tobacco. In combination, they significantly increase the risk of mouth, larynx, throat, esophagus, and liver cancers. According to some research, the synergistic action of heavy use of alcohol and tobacco yields a fifteen-fold increase in cancer of the oral cavity.

Maintenance of ideal body weight is also recommended. Obesity has been associated with colon, rectum, breast, prostate, gallbladder, ovary, and uterine cancers.

2. **Abstinence from cigarette smoking.** It has been reported that 83 percent of all lung cancer and 30 percent of all cancers are attributed to smoking. Smokeless tobacco also increases the risk of mouth, larynx, throat, and esophagus cancers. About 148,000 cancer deaths annually are attributed to the use of tobacco. The average life expectancy for a chronic smoker is seven years less than for a nonsmoker.

3. **Avoid sun exposure.** Sunlight exposure is a major factor in the development of skin cancer. Almost 100 percent of the 500,000 nonmelanoma skin cancer cases reported annually in the United States are related to sun exposure. Sun screen lotion should be used at all times when the skin is going to be exposed to sunlight for extended periods of time. Tanning of the skin is the body's natural reaction to cell damage taking place as a result of excessive sun exposure.

4. **Avoid estrogen use, radiation exposure, and occupational hazard exposure.** Estrogen use has been linked to endometrial cancer but can be taken safely under careful physician supervision. Radiation exposure also increases

cancer risk. Many times, however, the benefits of X-ray use outweigh the risk involved, and most medical facilities use the lowest dose possible to decrease the risk to a minimum. Occupational hazards, such as asbestos fibers, nickel and uranium dusts, chromium compounds, vinyl chloride, bis-chlormethyl ether, etc., increase cancer risk. The risk of occupational hazards is significantly magnified by the use of cigarette smoking.

Equally important is the fact that through early detection, many cancers can be controlled or cured. The real problem is the spreading of cancerous cells. Once spreading occurs, it becomes very difficult to wipe the cancer out. It is therefore crucial to practice effective prevention or at least catch cancer when the possibility of cure is greatest. Herein lies the importance of proper periodic screening for prevention and/or early detection.

The following are the seven warning signals for cancer. Every individual should become familiar with these warning signals and bring them to the attention of a physician if any of them are present:

1. Change in bowel or bladder habits.

2. A sore that does not heal.

3. Unusual bleeding or discharge.

4. Thickening or lump in breast or elsewhere.

5. Indigestion or difficulty in swallowing.

6. Obvious change in wart or mole.

7. Nagging cough or hoarseness.

Scientific evidence and testing procedures for prevention and/or early detection of cancer do change. Results of current clinical and epidemiologic studies provide constant new information about cancer prevention and detection. The purpose of cancer prevention programs is to educate and guide individuals toward a lifestyle that will aid them in the prevention and/or early detection of malignancy. Treatment of cancer should always be left to specialized physicians and cancer clinics.

ACCIDENTS

Most people do not perceive accidents as being a health problem, but accidents are the third leading cause of death in the United States, affecting the total well-being of millions of Americans each year. Accident prevention and personal safety are also part of a health enhancement program aimed at achieving a higher quality of life. Proper nutrition, exercise, abstinence from cigarette smoking, and stress management are of little help if the person is involved in a disabling or fatal accident due to distraction, a single reckless decision, or not properly wearing safety seat belts.

Accidents do not just happen. We cause accidents and we are victims of accidents. Although some factors in life are completely beyond our control, such as earthquakes, tornadoes, or airplane crashes, more often than not, personal safety and accident prevention are a matter of common sense. A majority of accidents are the result of poor judgment and confused mental states. Accidents frequently happen when we are upset, not paying attention to the task with which we are involved, or by abusing alcohol and other drugs.

Alcohol abuse is the number one cause of all accidents. Statistics clearly show that alcohol intoxication is the leading cause of most fatal automobile accidents. Other drugs commonly abused in society alter feelings and perceptions, lead to mental confusion, and impair judgment and coordination, thereby greatly enhancing the risk for accidental morbidity and mortality.

CHRONIC OBSTRUCTIVE PULMONARY DISEASE

Chronic obstructive pulmonary disease (COPD) is a term used to describe an air flow limiting disease that includes chronic bronchitis, emphysema, and a reactive airway component similar to that of asthma. The incidence of COPD increases proportionally with cigarette smoking (or other forms of tobacco use) and exposure to certain types of industrial pollution. In the case of emphysema, genetic factors may also play a role.

▬ IN CONCLUSION

Keep in mind that adequate fitness and total well-being is a process and you need to put forth a constant and deliberate effort to achieve and maintain a higher quality of life. To make your journey easier, remember to enjoy yourself and have fun along the way. If you implement your program based on what you enjoy doing most, adhering to a new lifestyle will not be difficult.

Hopefully, taking part in this class will help you develop positive "addictions" that will carry on throughout life. If you participate regularly and apply many of the principles explained in this book, you will truly experience a "new quality of life." Once you "reach the top," you will know that there is no looking back. But, if you do not get there, you will never know what it is like. Improving the quality and most likely the longevity of your life is now in your hands. It may require persistence and commitment, but only you can take control of your lifestyle and thereby reap the wellness benefits.

Appendix A

Although exercise testing and exercise participation is relatively safe for most apparently healthy individuals under age forty-five, the reaction of the cardiovascular system to increased levels of physical activity cannot always be totally predicted. Consequently, there is a small but real risk of certain changes occurring during exercise testing or participation. Some of these changes may include abnormal blood pressure, irregular heart rhythm, fainting, and, in rare instances, a heart attack or cardiac arrest.

Therefore, it is imperative that you provide honest answers to this questionnaire. Exercise may be contraindicated under some of the conditions listed below; others may simply require special consideration. **If any of the conditions apply, consult your physician before you participate in an exercise program.** Also, promptly report to your instructor any exercise-related abnormalities that you may experience during regular exercise participation.

A. Have you ever had or do you now have any of the following conditions:

☐ 1. A myocardial infarction
☐ 2. Coronary artery disease
☐ 3. Congestive heart failure
☐ 4. Elevated blood lipids (cholesterol and triglycerides)
☐ 5. Chest pain at rest or during exertion
☐ 6. Shortness of breath
☐ 7. An abnormal resting or stress electrocardiogram
☐ 8. Uneven, irregular, or skipped heartbeats (including a racing or fluttering heart)
☐ 9. A blood embolism
☐ 10. Thrombophlebitis
☐ 11. Rheumatic heart fever
☐ 12. Elevated blood pressure
☐ 13. A stroke
☐ 14. Diabetes
☐ 15. A family history of coronary heart disease, syncope, or sudden death before age sixty
☐ 16. Any other heart problem that makes exercise unsafe

FIGURE A.1. Health History Questionnaire (continued on page 146)

B. Do you suffer from any of the following conditions:
- ☐ 1. Arthritis, rheumatism, or gout
- ☐ 2. Chronic low back pain
- ☐ 3. Any other joint, bone, or muscle problems
- ☐ 4. Any respiratory problems
- ☐ 5. Obesity (more than 30 percent overweight)
- ☐ 6. Anorexia
- ☐ 7. Bulimia
- ☐ 8. Mononucleosis
- ☐ 9. Any physical disability that could interfere with safe exercise participation

C. Do any of the following conditions apply:
- ☐ 1. Do you smoke cigarettes?
- ☐ 2. Are you taking any prescription medication?
- ☐ 3. Are you forty-five years or older?

D. Do you have any other concern regarding your ability to safely participate in an exercise program? If so, explain:

_____

_____

Student's Signature: _____ Date: _____

Reproduced with permission from Hoeger, W. W. K. *Lifetime Physical Fitness & Wellness: A Personalized Program.* Morton Publishing Company, 1989.

FIGURE A.1. Health History Questionnaire (continued)

Appendix B

Date: _____ Course: _____ Section: _____

Name: _____ Age: _____ Male or Female: M/F

Body Weight: _____ . _____

Fitness Component	Test Results	Fitness Standard	Fitness Classification
Cardiovascular Endurance	Time ___.___	VO₂ max. ___.___	_____
Muscular Strength/Endurance	Reps	% tile	
Bench-Jumps	_____	_____	_____
Chair-Dips/Mod. Push-Ups	_____	_____	_____
Abdominal Curl-Ups	_____	_____	_____
Average Percentile		_____	_____
Muscular Flexibility	Inches	% tile	
Modified Sit-and-Reach	_____	_____	_____
Body Rotation (R/L)	_____	_____	_____
Average Percentile		_____	_____
Body Composition	mm		
Chest/Triceps	_____		
Abdominal/Suprailium	_____		
Thigh	_____	% Fat	
Sum of Skinfolds	_____	_____	_____

FIGURE B.1. Personal Fitness Profile: Pre-Test

Date: _____ Course: _____ Section: _____

Name: _____ Age: _____ Male or Female: M/F

Body Weight: _____ . _____

Fitness Component	Test Results	Fitness Standard	Fitness Classification
Cardiovascular Endurance	Time ___.___	VO$_2$ max. ___.___	_____
Muscular Strength/Endurance	Reps	% tile	
Bench-Jumps	_____	_____	_____
Chair-Dips/Mod. Push-Ups	_____	_____	_____
Abdominal Curl-Ups	_____	_____	_____
Average Percentile		_____	_____
Muscular Flexibility	Inches	% tile	
Modified Sit-and-Reach	_____	_____	_____
Body Rotation (R/L)	_____	_____	_____
Average Percentile		_____	_____
Body Composition	mm		
Chest/Triceps	_____		
Abdominal/Suprailium	_____		
Thigh	_____	% Fat	
Sum of Skinfolds	_____	_____	_____

FIGURE B.2. Personal Fitness Profile: Post Test

References

American Cancer Society. *1989 Cancer Facts and Figures.* New York: The Society, 1989.

American Cancer Society. *Cancer Book.* New York: The Society, 1986.

American College of Sports Medicine. *Guidelines for Graded Exercise Testing and Exercise Prescription.* Philadelphia, PA: Lea and Febiger, 1986.

American Heart Association Committee on Exercise. *Exercise Testing and Training of Apparently Healthy Individuals: A Handbook for Physicians.* New York: The Association, 1972.

American National Red Cross. *Swimming and Aquatics Safety.* Washington, D.C.: The American Red Cross, 1981.

Bar-Or, O., H. M. Lundgreen, and E. R. Buskirk. "Heat Tolerance of Exercising Obese and Lean Women." *Journal of Applied Physiology 26:* 403-409, 1969.

Cooper, K. H. "A Means of Assessing Maximal Oxygen Intake." *JAMA 203:* 201-204, 1968.

Cooper, K. H. *The Aerobics Program for Total Well-Being.* New York: Mount Evans and Co., 1982.

Croisant, P. T. "Effects of a Water Exercise Program Upon the Fitness of Older Individuals." Abstracts: Research Papers 1986 AAHPERD Convention, 1986.

Christian, J. L. and J. L. Greger. *Nutrition for Living.* Menlo Park, CA: The Benjamin/Cummings Publishing Company, Inc., 1988.

Hoeger, W. W. K. *Lifetime Physical Fitness and Wellness: A Personalized Program.* Englewood, CO: Morton Publishing Company, 1989.

Hoeger, W. W. K. *Principles and Labs for Physical Fitness and Wellness.* Englewood, CO: Morton Publishing Company, 1988.

LeCompte, J. D., and S. Antony. "Water Exercise for the '90s." *Fitness Management 5:* 24-27.

Maglischo, E. W., and C. F. Brennan. *Swimming for the Health of It*. Palo Alto, CA: Mayfield Publishing Company, 1985.

McArdle, W. D., F. I. Katch, and V. L. Katch. *Exercise Physiology: Energy, Nutrition and Human Performance*. Philadelphia, PA: Lea and Febiger, 1986.

Morgan, B. L. G. *The Lifelong Nutrition Guide*. Englewood Cliffs, NJ: Prentice- Hall, 1983.

Pollock, M. L., J. H. Wilmore and S. M. Fox III. *Health and Fitness Through Physical Activity*. New York: John Wiley & Sons, 1978.

VanGelder, N. and S. Marks. *Aerobic Dance-Exercise Instructor Manual*. San Diego, CA: International Dance-Exercise Association (IDEA) Foundation, 1987.

Whitney, E. N. and E. V. N. Hamilton. *Understanding Nutrition*. St. Paul, MN: West Publishing Co., 1987.

Wilmore, J. H. *Training for Sport and Activity*. Boston, MA: Allyn and Bacon, Inc., 1982.

Index

abdomen
  and body fat assessment, 30
abnormalities, cardiac, 46
accidents, 132, 143
acid-base balance, 113
Acuflex I, 21
Acuflex II, 24, 25
"addictions," positive, 144
adipose tissue, 3, 29
  and flexibility, 20
aerobic capacity, 10
aerobic dance, iii, 5, 45, 124
aerobic phase, 41, 43–47
  objectives of, 43
  parts of, 46
aerobic program, 123
  and cholesterol, 136
Aerobics Research Center, 124
age, 139
aging, 7
  and flexibility, 20
airborne jumping jacks, 83
alcohol, 1, 7, 111, 114, 132, 140, 141, 143
alcoholism
  and diet, 115
amenorrhea, 118, 119
American Cancer Society, 140
American Medical Association, 2
American Heart Association, 135
American, "typical," 10
anatomical landmarks
  for skinfolds, 30
anemia, 118
ankle circles, 97
anorexia nervosa, 117–119
antibodies, 113
aortic aneurysm, 138
appearance, physical, 6, 13
  and flexibility, 20, 52
appendicitis, 112
arm across, 104
arm circles, forward and back, 63
arms in, arms out, 38
arrhythmias
  and bulimia, 119
  and smoking, 138
arthritis, 5, 7
artificial sweeteners, 123
asbestos
  and cancer, 142
assessment, of exercise program, 53
atherosclerosis, 28, 134, 136, 138
attitude, toward fitness, 41
"automatic" eating, 126

back lift, 103
back problems, 52
back strain, 64
ball of foot, 37
bench-jumps, 15, 15

bent-leg curl-ups, 17, 18
bicep curls, 70
biceps-curl, 35
bicycles, 98
binge eating, 118
bischlormethyl ether
  and cancer, 142
bladder
  changes in, 142
  damage to, 119
blood pressure, 10
  intercostal, 49
blood vessels, 11
body builders, 28
body composition, 3, 27–32, 32
  ideal, 123, 125, 135, 136
body fluid balance, 113
body temperature
  and flexibility, 20
body weight, ideal, 6, 141
  determination of, 32
bones
  and stress, 5
boredom
  and eating habits, 126
bowel, changes in, 142
breast cancer, 29
bulimia, 117–119
buoyancy effect, 36
  and pull buoys, 50

cadence
  for water aerobics music, 38
calcium, 40
calipers, pressure, 29, 30
calisthenics, 20, 52
calories, 14, 111, 113–117, 122
can can, 67
cancer, 112, 138, 140–142
  definition of, 140
  prevention, 132, 140–142
  warning signals for, 142
cannonball, 82
carbohydrates, 10, 111–114, 123, 124
cardiac muscle strength, 10
cardiovascular development, 4
cardiovascular disease. See heart disease
cardiovascular endurance. See endurance
cardiovascular fitness
  classification, 13
cardiovascular risk reduction, 132–139
cardiovascular system, 6, 43, 45, 132
  and obesity, 28
carotid artery, 44, 46
cassette players, battery-charged, 38

cells, maintenance of, 112
cellulite, 124
chair-dips, 16, 16
chart, goal-setting, 41, 42
cheerleader jump, 80
chest
  and body fat assessment, 29, 30
  discomfort and stress ECG, 137
childbirth, 7
cholesterol, 10, 134–136
  levels of, 135–137
  types of (HDL, LDL), 136
chromium
  and cancer, 142
chronic bronchitis, 138, 143
"chronic exerciser," 53
chronic obstructive pulmonary disease, 132, 143
chronotropic incompetence, 137
chylomicrons, 137
circulatory system, 10, 132
claudication, intermittent, 28
climb the wall, 73
cocoa butter, 136
colitis, ulcerative, 112, 119
commitment, to change, 125
confusion, 118
congenital heart disease, 132
congestive heart failure, 133
  and obesity, 28
constipation, 112
cooking, for weight management, 127
cool-down, 20, 53
  aerobic, 46
Cooper, Kenneth H., 135
coronary heart disease, 1
  and obesity, 28, 132
  risk factors for, 134–139
cough
  and cancer, 142
cramps, muscle, 40
cross country skier, 77
"cushioning" effect, 5, 37
cycling, stationary, 41, 45, 124, 126

deep water cross country, 86
deep water job, 86
delivery. See pregnancy
depression, 7, 118
  and eating habits, 126
dextrins, 112
diabetics
  and stress ECGs, 137
diet
  balanced, 113–117
  fad, 119
  low-calorie, 115
  low-salt, 135
  typical American, 111
dieting, 29

digestive difficulties, 118
discomfort
 and exercise, 40, 60
diseases, chronic, 1, 7
diverticulitis, 112
dizziness, 46
donkey kick, 84
downward hugs, 72
drag force, 34, 35
drugs, 1, 7
dryness, skin, 118
duration, of exercise, 45
dysmennorhea, 20, 52
dysrhythmias
 and stress ECG, 137

eating disorders, 117–119. See also
 individual listings
eating habits
 healthy, 126
 retraining of, 123
education, health, 132, 140
eggbeater, 76
egg consumption, 132
elbow to knee, 74
elderly, the, 5
electrocardiogram (ECG), 135
 stress, 137
electrolytes, 40
 abnormalities, 119
emetics,
 and bulimia, 118
emphysema 138, 143
endurance
 cardiovascular, 2, 34, 46
  and heart disease, 135
  assessment, 10–13
  definition of, 14
  determination of, 10
 muscular, 2, 5, 6, 34, 48
  assessment, 13–20
  scoring table, 19
  test, muscular, 14
environmental management, for
 weight management, 128
enzymes, 113
 fat-burning, 124
esophagus, damage to, 119
estrogen, use of, 141
exercise
 bench-jumps, 15, 15, 19
 bent-leg curl-ups, 17, 18, 19
 chair-dips, 16, 16
 flexibility, 43
 isolation, 43
 jumping, 5
 locomotor, 5
 modified push-ups, 16, 17, 19
 strength-training, 20
 warm-up, 43
exercise program, lifetime, 123
 and exercise, 126
exercises, for water aerobics,
 54–110. See also individual
 listings for each exercise
 list of exercises, 57–59
 tips for, 60
extremities, upper and lower, 5

failure, 129
faintness, 46
family history, 139
fast foods, 115
fat, 48
 determination of percentage in
  diet, 114
 essential, 29
 sex-specific, 29
 storage, 29, 120–121
 subcutaneous, 29
fatigue, 53
fat mass, 3, 28
fats, 10, 111–112
 saturated, 114, 123
fatty acids, 112, 137
fatty foods, 1, 132
fatty tissue, 14
fiber, 111, 112, 114
 importance of, 112
 sources of, 112
Figure 8, 88
fitness, physical
 assessment of, 9–31
 categories based on percentile
  ranks, 20
 components of, 2, 2, 9–32
 definition of, 2
 goals, 43, 42, 53
 programs, iii, 1, 2, 33–110
 tests, 9–32
flexibility, 2, 6, 20–28, 34, 41,
 52–53
 assessment, 20–28
 definition of, 20
 exercises, 43
 tests, 21–28
flutter kicks, 96
food management, 124
foods, refined, 112
football players
 and body composition, 28
frequency, of exercise, 45
froggies, 80
fun, 60

gallbladder disease, 112
gardening, 126
gender
 and flexibility, 20
glucose, 124
goals, See fitness
goal-setting, realistic, 125–126
golfer, 88
"good" cholesterol, 136
"good life," 1
gums, damage to, 119

habit
 and eating patterns, 126
habits, modification of, 125–129
hamstring wall stretch, 107
hand paddles, 49–50, 50, 60
 precautions for use, 49–50
hand position, in water, 35, 36,
 54, 60
hand squeezes, 92
head down exercise, 61
head turn exercise, 61

health history questionnaire,
 145–146
heat, 5, 6, 37
heat exhaustion, 6, 38
heat stress, 6, 38
heat stroke, 6
heart, 10
heartbeat, irregular, 118
heart disease, 7, 11, 112, 132–139
heart muscle, 43
heart rate, 10, 43–45, 54
 maximal, 44
 range, 46
 reserve, 44
 resting, 44
heel touches, 66
height/weight charts, 28
hemorrhoids, 112
high blood pressure, 7, 132, 133
high-density lipoprotein
 cholesterol. See cholesterol
hip flexor stretch, 109
hoarseness
 and cancer, 142
hormones, 113
housework
 and muscular strength, 13, 48
hugs, 87
hypertension, 1, 135
 and stress ECG, 137
hypokinetic diseases, 10

immune function, 118
inactivity
 and health, 1
Indian, 105
indigestion
 and cancer, 142
individualization, of exercise, 40,
 48, 54
infants
 and vitamin supplementation,
  115
injuries, athletic, 5
 overuse, 48
 prevention of, 39–41, 43
 to the back, 38
 twisting action and, 39
intensity, of exercise, 35, 39, 40,
 43–45, 47, 54
Irish jig, 74
iron, deficiency, 115
isolation exercises, 43

job productivity, 7
jogging, iii, 5, 11, 45, 124
jogging hugs, 71
joints, 2, 3, 5, 35, 39, 60
 impact on, 56
 injuries to, 124
 protection of, 50
 range of motion, 38, 43, 47, 52,
  60
 structure, 20
jumping jack, 68
jump rope, 85
"junk" food, 112

kick-up front, 84
kidneys, damage to, 119

knee lifts, 43, *64*
knee, problems with, *64*
knee to chest, *108*

lactation
    and diet, 115
    and water exercise, 40
"lat" pull, *81*
laxatives
    and bulimia, 118
lean body mass, 3, 14, 28, 29, 122, 123
leaps, *69*
leg front and backs, *95*
leg lifts, *65*
leg pendulum, *95*
length, of exercising limb, 35
lethargy, 118
Level I exercises, 54
Level II exercises, 54
Level III exercises, 54
levers, 35, 47, 54, 60
lifestyle, healthy, iii, 1
lifestyle, negative, 131
lifting, 48
ligaments
    and flexibility, 20
    and stress, 5
limb movement
    motion in water, 39
    speed of in water, 34–35
    tempo of, 47
lipids, blood, 10, 135–137
    and obesity, 28
    as source of energy, 112
liver, 136, 137
longevity, 131
low-density lipoprotein
    cholesterol (LDL). *See*
    cholesterol
lumps
    and cancer, 142
lungs, 10

macronutrients, 111
maximal amount of resistance, 14
meal planning, 126
meats, organ, 136
meats, red, 136
menstruation
    and vitamin supplementation, 115
metabolic imbalance
    and diet, 119
metabolic rate, 48
metabolism, energy, 6, 14, 113
    definition of, 14
micronutrients, 111
milk jug ankle circles, *100*
milk jug bicycles, *101*
milk jug flutters, *99*
milk jug leg scissors, *98*
milk jug quad and hams, *101*
milk jugs, 49, 51–52, *52*, *60*
milk jug strides, *99*
milk jug toe taps, *100*
minerals, 111
mode, of exercise, 43, 45
modified push-ups, 16, *17*

modified sit-and-reach test, 21, *22*, *23*
moles
    and cancer, 142
monitoring, of changes, 128
motivation, 125–126
motor skills
    and flexibility, 20
movement
    and flexibility, 20
muscle, injuries to, 124
muscle tissue, 14
    and flexibility, 20
muscular endurance. *See*
    endurance
muscular strength. *See* strength
musculo-skeletal problems, iii, 33
    and flexibility, 20
music
    during aerobics class, 38

neck and double arm stretch, *107*
neck, injury to, *61*
neck presses, *87*
neuromuscular tension, 20, 52
nickel
    and cancer, 142
nomogram for percent fat
    determination, *31*
"no pain, no gain" philosophy, 47
nutrient density
    high, 112
    low, 112
nutrition, 7, 111–129, 132

obesity, 5, 6, 28, 112
objectives, short-term, 126
occupational hazards, 140, 141
oil
    coconut, 136
    palm, 136
overconsumption
    of fat, 114
    of food, 111
overexercising, 53
overload, 47, 49
overload principle, 34, 35, 48
overuse injuries. *See* injuries
oxygen, 10–11
oxygen-carrying capacity, 10
oxygen uptake, 11, *12*, 13

pacing
    and exercise, 47
paddle position. *See* hand position
paddles, hand. *See* hand paddles
pain
    and exercise, 40, 60
parallel arms, *77*
pendulum arms, *73*
pendulums, *89*
percent body fat, 28, 123
    reduction in, 124
performance
    and nutrition, 111
peripheral vascular disease, 132
physical activity
    and flexibility, 20
pollution
    and COPD, 143

pool bottom, 37
pool depth
    and milk jugs, 52
pool surface, 36
positive thinking, 128
posture, 6
    and alignment, 52
    and flexibility, 20
pregnancy
    and diet, 115
    and water exercise, 40–41
press downs, *70*
pre-stretches, 43, 44
prevention, of chronic diseases, 2
protein, 111, 113, 114
pull buoy, 49, 50–51, *51*, *60*
pulmonary disease, 7
pulse, 46–47
purging
    and bulimia, 119
pushdown jump, *78*
pushdown stride, *79*
push-ups, *90*

quad stretch, *103*
quality of life, 3, 7, 131

racquetball, 45
radial artery, 44, 46
radiation, exposure to, 141
raids, on refrigerator and cookie
    jar, 128
range of motion. *See* joints
rate, exercise. *See* pulse
rear leg lifts, *64*
recovery time, 7, 10, 41
Red Cross, 39
repetition maximum, 14
repetitions, 48
reserve capacity, of the heart, 44
resistance, 33, 34, 36, 47, 48, 50
rewards, for accomplishment, 128
rheumatic heart disease, 132
risk factors
    for cancer, 132
    for cerebro-vascular disease, 132
    for heart disease, 132
rockers, *85*
rope skipping, 45
rotator cuff, *93*
roughage. *See* fiber
row the boat, *81*
running, 48. *See also* jogging
run/walk test, 1.5-mile, 11, *12*
    cautions for, 11
    contraindications for, 11
    warm-up exercises for, 11
Russian, the *68*

safe environment
    and water aerobics, 3
seat belts, 132, 143
sedentary living, 1, 10, 29
self-confidence, lack of, 118
self-image, 7, 13, 20, 52
sensitivity, to cold, 118
servings, minimum number of,
    117, *116*
sequence, of exercise
    sample, *55–56*

set, definition of, 49
shellfish, 136
shoulder circles, *62*
shoulder depressions, *106*
shoulder girdle exercise
　depressions, *62*
　elevations, *62*
shoulder muscles, 38
side leg lift, *94*
side lift, *105*
sit-and-reach box, 21
sitting, 48
skater, *75*
skiing, cross-country, 45
skin
　and flexibility, 20
skinfold thickness, 29
"skinny"
　and body composition, 29
smoking, 7, 138
　and stress ECG, 137
　cessation, 132, 135, 141, 143
social binges, 126
socialization
　and water aerobics, 3
sodium, 111, 114
sores
　and cancer, 142
spinal column problems
　and flexibility, 20
sports skills, 13
spot reducing, 124
squeezes, *90*
stair climbing, 45
standing calf stretch, *102*
standing hamstring, *102*
starches, 112
starvation, 117, 118
straight jump, *79*
strength improvement
　and water aerobics, 3
strength, muscular, 2, 6, 13–20,
　34, 48
　definition of, 14
strength-training program, 123
stress, 7, 126, 128, 132, 138–139
stretching exercises, 11
stroke, 1, 7, 28, 133, 138
submaximal resistance, 14
substance abuse, control of, 132
sudden death, 134, 138
sugars, 111–112, 122, 123
sunlight, exposure to, 140, 141
supplementation
　mineral, 115–116
　vitamin, 115–116
suprailium
　and body fat assessment, 29, 30
surface area, 49, 60
sweets, 1, 114
swimsuits, 38–39
swimming, 45
syncope
　and stress ECG, 137

tailor, *110*
talking, during exercise, 47
target heart rate zone, 35,
　43–45, 46, 48

target training zone. *See* target
　heart rate zone
temperature
　of air, 43
　of water, 37, 43, 53
tempo
　and exercise, 47, 54, 60, *70*
　with pull buoys, 51
tendons
　and flexibility, 20
　and impact, 36
　and stress, 5
tension. *See* stress
thigh
　and body fat assessment, 29, 30
thromboembolitic disease, 28
tissue injury
　and flexibility, 20
tobacco, 1, 132, 140. *See also*
　smoking
toe jogs, *65*
toe taps, *97*
tone, muscular, 6
toning, 35, 41, 47, 53
　phase, 48–52
　special equipment for, 49–52
tooth, erosion, 119
torso rotation, *63*
total body rotation test, 24, *25,*
　26, 27
training zone, 38
tricep, *104*
tricep kickbacks, *89*
triceps
　and body fat assessment, 29, 30
triglycerides, 10, 134, 135, 136, 137
　and very low-density
　　lipoproteins (VLDL), 137
tumors, 140
　benign, 140
　malignant, 140
twisting actions, *60*

ulcers, 119, 138
uranium
　and cancer, 142
uterus, 29

valsalva maneuver, 49
varicose veins, 28
vegetables, cruciferous, 140–141
vegetarianism
　and vitamin supplementation,
　　115
vertigo, 61
very low-density lipoprotein. *See*
　triglycerides
vinyl chloride
　and cancer, 142
vitamins, 111–113
　fat-soluble, 112
　water-soluble, 113
vomiting
　and bulimia, 119

walking, 11, 41, 45, 124, 126
　in water, 34
wall arm stretch, *106*

wall calf stretch, *108*
wall curls, *94*
wall scissors, *96*
wall straddle, *110*
warm-up phase, 41, 43, 53
　exercises for, 43
warts
　and cancer, 142
water, as a nutrient, 111
water
　buoyancy of, 5
　characteristics of, 5
　density of, 5
　resistance of, 5
water aerobics
　advantages of, 4–6
　arms in vs. arms out issue, 38
　benefits of, 6–7
　exercises for, 54–110
　fitness program, 33–110
　history of, 4
　number of participants in, 3
　pool surface for, 36
　principles of, 34–35
　purpose of, 41
　special considerations for, 36–39
　special tips for, 38–39
　temperature of water, 37
　water depth for, 36, *37*
　what it provides, 3
water balance
　and nutrition, 113
water depth, 36, *37*
weakness, muscular, 119
weight control, principles of,
　119–123
weight, fat, 123
weight, ideal, 119
　and bulimia, 118
weight lift, *82*
weight lifters, 28
weight management, lifetime,
　125–129
weight reduction, 3, 48
wellness, 7
　approach to life, 131
　components of, 132, *133*
　definition of, 131–132
wet-vest, 86
window wash, *91*
workout, aerobic, 46
wrist circles, *92*

X-rays
　and cancer, 142

YMCA, 39
YWCA, 39